'General practice has long been the jewel in the crown of the UK National Health Service; *A Fortunate Woman* sets out in compelling detail the relationship-based care that will be lost forever if we do not act to support and revitalise a profession under threat. It is a vibrant and authentic portrait of the rural family doctor in these difficult contemporary times.'

**Trisha Greenhalgh, Professor of Primary Care
at the University of Oxford**

'This beautifully crafted book drew me in immediately by reminding me of so many reasons why I became a General Practitioner in the first place – relationship-based care and truly holistic practice. *A Fortunate Woman* is grounded in a legacy of care and compassion for the community served, shared through a compelling narrative based on patient stories. I loved it.'

**Professor Dame Helen Stokes-Lampard,
Chair of the Academy of Medical Colleges**

'Stunning in style and content and I hope it encourages all readers to reflect on its key message – the importance of relationship-based care and the fact that it is under threat.'

**Professor Martin Marshall, former Chair of
the Royal College of General Practitioners**

First published 2022 by Picador

This paperback edition published 2023 by Picador
an imprint of Pan Macmillan
The Smithson, 6 Briset Street, London EC1M 5NR
EU representative: Macmillan Publishers Ireland Ltd, 1st Floor,
The Liffey Trust Centre, 117–126 Sheriff Street Upper,
Dublin 1, DO1 YC43
Associated companies throughout the world
www.panmacmillan.com

ISBN 978-1-5290-7117-7

1 3 5 7 9 8 6 4 2

A CIP catalogue record for this book is available from the British Library.

Printed and bound by CPI Group (UK) Ltd, Croydon, CR0 4YY

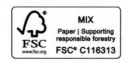

'Morland writes about nature and the changing landscape with such lyrical precision that her prose sometimes seems close to poetry . . . There has been no shortage in recent years of books about healthcare . . . With this gem, Morland has done something similar for general practice. Let's just hope the policymakers listen.'

Christina Patterson, *The Sunday Times*

'Superb – beautiful, enthralling, careful, tender, a humanitarian act in itself, deeply moral, moving, lucid and loving.'

Laura Cumming, James Tait Black winner and bestselling Costa-shortlisted author of *The Vanishing Man* and *On Chapel Sands*

'The descriptions of both the people and the place are a delight, beautifully illustrated by Richard Baker's photographs. Although there is loss and grief in this book, it is also a celebration of what general practice can be at its best. Recommended reading for all aspiring doctors, and especially for those working in health policy, so they may understand and preserve the crown jewels of the NHS.'

Dr Helen Salisbury, Senior Medical Education Fellow, Nuffield Department of Primary Care Health Sciences, University of Oxford

'One of the best books about medicine that I have read. The patients' stories are vivid, moving, often unforgettable. Polly Morland has written with incredible sensitivity, appreciation and descriptive ability about the valley and the people who live there.'

Professor Roger Jones OBE

'Beautifully and tenderly written, [*A Fortunate Woman*] also serves as a topical reminder of what is possible with continuity of care.'

Caroline Sanderson, 'Editor's Choice',
The Bookseller

'Here is inbuilt drama, the tug of emotion, self-sacrifice and community, all topped with the glisten of protruding bones and accompanied by howls of anguish.'

The Times

'All human life is here in this evocative portrayal of the challenges and joys of rural family doctoring in modern times. Enthralling and uplifting.'

James LeFanu, author of
The Rise & Fall of Modern Medicine

'*A Fortunate Woman* is the best book I've read about general practice for a long time. Astonishingly perceptive, it shows how a committed GP can keep human values alive in an increasingly impersonal NHS – and why we urgently need more like her.'

Professor Roger Neighbour OBE, past President,
Royal College of General Practitioners

A Fortunate Woman

Polly Morland is a writer and documentary maker. She worked for fifteen years in television, producing and directing documentaries for the BBC, Channel 4 and Discovery. She is a regular contributor to newspapers and magazines and is the Royal Literary Fund Fellow in the School of Journalism, Media & Culture at Cardiff University. She is the author of several books, including *The Society of Timid Souls: Or, How to Be Brave*, which was shortlisted for the *Guardian* First Book Award and was a *Sunday Times* Book of the Year. *A Fortunate Woman* was shortlisted for the Baillie Gifford Prize for Non-Fiction 2022.

POLLY MORLAND

A Fortunate Woman

A Country Doctor's Story

With photographs by Richard Baker

PICADOR

This book is dedicated to R.

whom it concerns,

& to Pat Williams (1931–2020),

who lit the spark.

Now the patient is the central character.

– JOHN BERGER, *A Fortunate Man*

Prologue

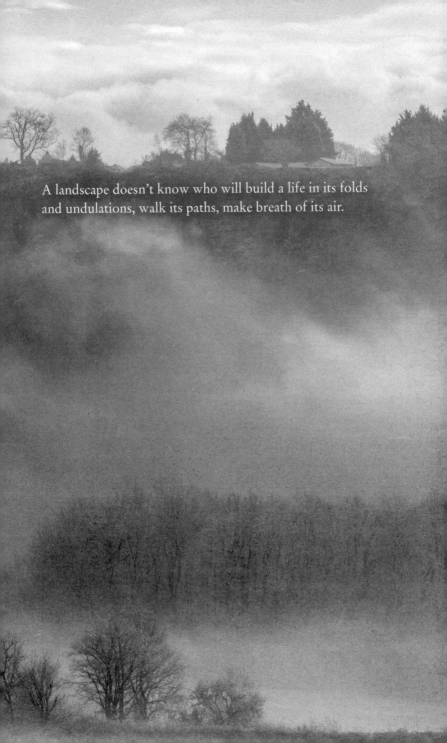

A landscape doesn't know who will build a life in its folds and undulations, walk its paths, make breath of its air.

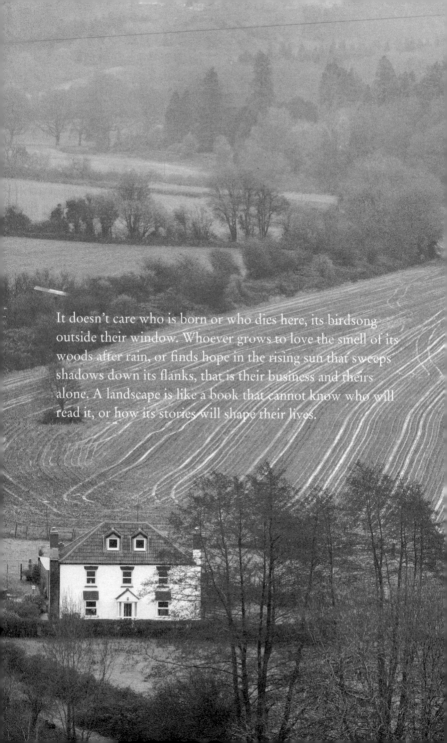

It doesn't care who is born or who dies here, its birdsong outside their window. Whoever grows to love the smell of its woods after rain, or finds hope in the rising sun that sweeps shadows down its flanks, that is their business and theirs alone. A landscape is like a book that cannot know who will read it, or how its stories will shape their lives.

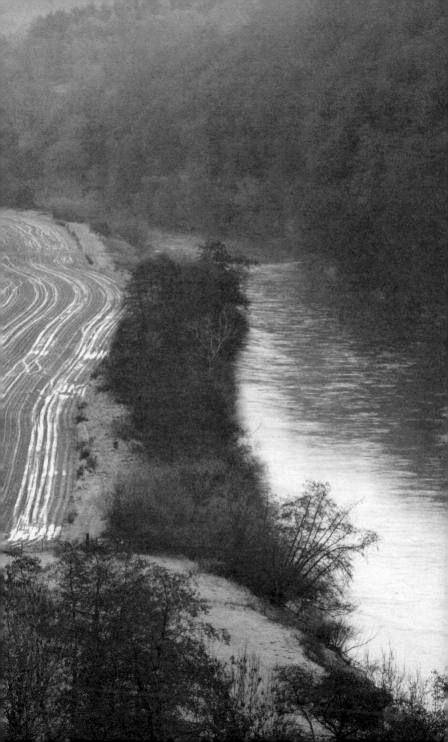

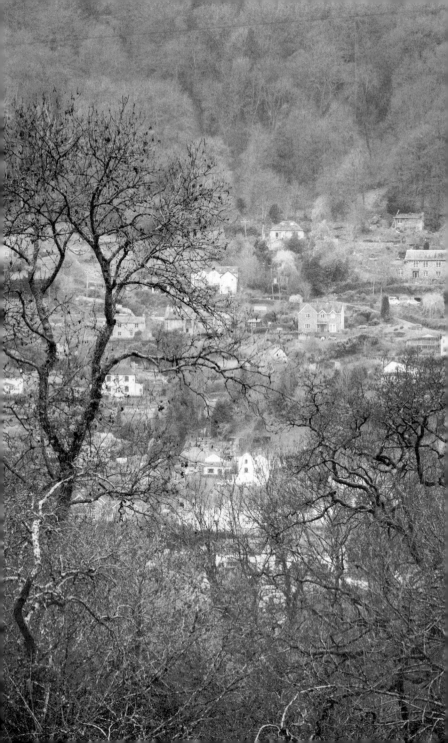

I FOUND A BOOK, unopened for nearly fifty years. It had fallen behind my parents' bookshelves half a lifetime ago, but never hit the floor, instead hanging in suspended animation, looped on a metal strut mid-air. An old Penguin paperback of John Berger's *A Fortunate Man*, priced at 45 new pence or 9 shillings.

It was the summer of 2020 and I was clearing out my parents' house. My father was long dead and my mother, then in her eighties, was suffering from Alzheimer's. Her last year here had been frightening and chaotic, filled with a succession of doctors and paramedics, nurses and social workers, all well meaning and professional, but none of whom had known my mother before all this started, nor stayed long enough to get to know her now. A string of hospital stays followed, culminating in a bout of Covid-19. Finally, she was transferred from an acute elderly ward, where the virus was taking hold, into a care home. So now the house she and my father had shared must be emptied and sold.

Surrounded by boxes, packing cases, and all the debris of a long life, I fished the paperback out from behind the shelves and smoothed the dust from it. First published in 1967, this edition was from 1971, which meant, I realized, that my mother had bought *A Fortunate Man* when she was pregnant with me. '*The Story of a Country Doctor*' it said on the cover. Below was a black-and-white photo, blurry with movement, of a man in shirtsleeves, a pair of long, curved forceps in each hand, the outline of a patient lying on a bed behind him. I turned to the opening page, where I was startled by a photograph that spanned the double spread.

The image shows a river, its banks thick with rough grass, rising to a broad field fringed by hedgerows. A single handsome oak in full leaf draws the eye upwards to the valley sides, inky with dense woodland, beneath a flat, pale English sky. Silhouetted in the morning light, two men are fishing from a small skiff, one at the oars, the other rod in hand. Their reflections in the river are mirror-sharp between eddies and mazy patches that hint at the current beneath.

I knew that river, that field. I knew that tree. As I'd left home early that morning to drive the hundred and fifty miles to my mother's house in the Midlands, I could have taken just such a photograph myself.

Standing there, knee-deep in our family ephemera, I scanned the pages for familiar place names and found none. So I tapped the title of the book into my phone. Sure enough, *A Fortunate Man* takes place in the same remote, rural valley that's been my home for the last decade. The book is an account of six weeks in 1966 that the critic and writer John Berger, and the photographer Jean Mohr, spent documenting the work of the local doctor.

It was this that made my heart skip a beat. For not only was this my home, my valley, but I too knew the doctor, his successor, the woman who serves this same community today. I knew she was a similar age to me, a similar age to this book I was holding. I knew she'd spent twenty years at the medical practice with its twin surgeries up on each shoulder of the valley. I knew that people trust her and that she loves her job, rarely takes a day off. I knew people said it's unusual nowadays to have a family doctor like her, almost as if she were some trace of a bygone age. A fortunate woman like her predecessor, perhaps, but then – my next thought – *God, what a time to be a doctor.*

Of this I was certain: something had aligned, urgent and irresistible; something connecting these highly medicalized and strangely impersonal months in my beloved mother's life and the book I found, by chance, in the home she'd had to leave; something connecting the author of the book and me, a place, a landscape, a story; above all, something that bound fast the physician pictured on the cover of the paperback in my hand and a woman I know today, an ordinary doctor who walks in his footsteps. I wasn't yet sure how or why, but these things seemed threaded together – as a river threads through a landscape.

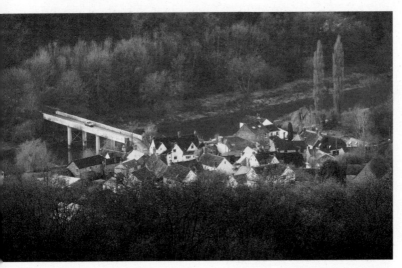

A FORTUNATE MAN never names the locality in which it is set, nor identifies the doctor's patients whose stories are told. 'None of the case histories in this book,' reads the copyright page, 'refer to particular persons; each has been compounded from several cases.' Even the name 'Dr John Sassall' is a pseudonym. Rather than a piece of journalism per se, Berger sifted the fine detail of this country doctor's life and his valley community, panning it like river silt for gold. The resulting meditation on the nature of the doctor–patient relationship framed 'Sassall' as a paragon of empathy and dedication, and it made the book a classic, albeit an obscure one. To this day, A Fortunate Man remains much loved by doctors, oft quoted in medical literature and a fixture on trainee medics' reading lists.

Still, for all its seminal importance, the world has turned in the half century since *A Fortunate Man* was written. Medicine is different. Rural life is different. Society, class, gender, all radically transformed since the 1960s. Doctors are different too, not least in the fact that, certainly in primary care, now well over half of them are women. Quite apart from the pandemic that was in full flow, didn't my chance discovery, this unwitting gift from my mother, present an opportunity, an obligation, to revisit this tale of a country doctor with a fresh gaze?

I set aside the book, emailed the doctor and, within the hour, she'd replied. Yes, she knew the book. Yes, it had played an extraordinary part in her own story; she'd explain how. And yes, yes, we should meet. If the weather was fine, she wrote, we could sit and talk on the old pew salvaged by the parish sexton during the renovation of the village church and positioned on a hummock in the wet meadow behind the surgery. So this is how we began, the doctor and I, amid marsh orchids, wood anemones and birdsong.

THE STORY THAT FOLLOWS pieced itself together over the next twelve months. Our first meeting by the meadow came during the lull after the first wave of the Covid pandemic, and it wasn't long before another wave rolled in. Through necessity, over-the-shoulder observation gave way to conversation. GPs are taught that they need to listen, she said, so it's unusual to talk. Yet it was exactly this that opened up the story far beyond the emergency of the moment. We'd walk, for hours at a time, through the woods of the valley, head torches bent on the winter-dark path, or as the months passed, the forest floor dappled by shafts of spring sunshine where the doctor's dogs bustled at our feet. As we walked, she told me about her life, what it is and what it means to be a doctor in a place like this, at a time like this.

It was not that she was out of the ordinary; she needed me to understand that. In many ways, she was like any hard-working GP, except for the turn of good fortune that had brought her to this valley, this practice, this community. For such is the nature of the landscape here and the people for whom it is home, that it shapes, indeed demands, a form of medical practice that is fast disappearing, as my mother and I knew all too well. Put simply, she is a doctor who knows her patients. She is the keeper of their stories, over years and across generations, witness to the infinite variety of their lives. These stories, she says, are what her job is all about. They are what sustains her, even in days as hard as these.

This is a true account. Everything in the pages that follow transpired in some form, at some time, during the doctor's working life. However, the confidentiality of the medical consultation is sacrosanct, protected both by ethical obligation and by law. That's why the details of specific patient consultations have been reimagined and reconfigured into composites, so as to be unrecognizable. In all but three stories, where anonymity would have been impossible to preserve and where patient consent was given, no case history relates to a single individual. Periodically, when lockdown permitted, we were joined in the valley by a long-time collaborator of mine, the photographer Richard Baker. It should be noted that no patients who appear in his photographs bear any correspondence to the stories told. Maintaining confidentiality has remained of the utmost importance throughout the process. This, so the doctor explained, was the only way she could truly show the relationships at the heart of her work. 'I love this job very much,' she wrote to me before our first long walk together, 'so my patients' trust is more important to me than anything I can think of.'

And that seems a fitting place to begin.

He limps into the room, trailing a faint tang of sheep.

'Morning.' The word comes out a single syllable. He lowers himself, with a sharp, tinny exhalation, into the chair by the desk, which creaks under his weight. He is one of those patients not given to troubling the doctor with minor ailments. She masks the concern his presence causes with a few pleasantries about the damp weather. Then she rolls her seat back from the desk to face him and, assuming the comfortable posture, hands folded in lap, that she's learned puts her patients at ease, she asks how she can help today.

'My chest, doctor.' He pauses. 'Rattling cough. Can't seem to shift.' She asks to take a look at his throat and listen to his chest. A mouthful of fillings yawns wide, his eyes turned to the wall. As he unbuttons the checked flannel of his shirt for the cold stethoscope, the doctor asks after his wife, says she's glad when she hears that Mary is 'much better and all that'. But the man is not smiling. The doctor watches his face and listens, first on one side of his barrel chest, then on the other. His breathing sounds as old men's lungs do when they've spent a lifetime around hay, straw and chemical sheep dip, wheezy, but not unusually so.

'It was the wife suggest I come down here.'

His face is greyer than it usually is when she passes him in his pickup on the lanes. Mary was perhaps worried about something, she says, helping him remove one sleeve and stepping behind an expanse of whiskery back. He doesn't reply, but she can see an uncomfortable stillness in his shoulders. She positions the stethoscope, listens left and right.

'Course if it's nothing' – he moves both hands to the arms of the chair and makes to get up – 'I'll be off.'

She touches his shoulder to stop him and now the doctor is playing for time. Asking how things are up on the hill, she checks his blood pressure, pulse, temperature. She has often said, and only half in jest, that farmers are always richer and sharper than they appear. She doesn't see so many of them these days. Truth is, she admires an intelligence moulded outside of conventional education and, although it doesn't make her job any easier, she is moved by the old-world stoicism of their way of life. It makes her think of the wind on the lip of the valley and how it has crooked the branches of the trees that grow there to withstand even the wildest weather. She knows an A&E doctor at a nearby hospital who won't let any farmer be discharged without first being reviewed by a consultant; the very fact they're there is usually an indication that something's seriously wrong. Now, as the man shrugs his bulk back into his shirt, she mentions the limp she noticed when he arrived. You don't usually limp, she says, and asks if he's in pain. She uses his first name, meets his eye. He shrugs, almost imperceptibly. 'S'pose I am, doctor.' He has instinctively cupped his palm at the top of his right thigh. 'Tussle with a gate the other day.'

Piece by piece, she draws the story out. The said tussle took place two weeks ago. The pain has remained ever since. One leg feels shorter than the other. He'll need an X-ray, she says, to rule out hairline fractures.

'But we're lambing. Another couple of hundred ewes to go, so.' She pictures the lambing shed, folded into an envelope of woodland half a mile along the ridge out of the village, and she asks how he's managing to lamb with that painful leg.

'I crawl.'

He pauses. She waits.

'After she's lambed, the ewe, I just, you know, hands and knees over to the quad and use the little ladder there on the side to pull myself up.' He looks her directly in the eye, this schoolgirl who's been his doctor these twenty years. 'Not the end of the world, doctor.'

She wheels her chair back to the computer on the desk and, kind but firm, makes an X-ray appointment two hours from now up at the forest hospital, checking he can get there without an ambulance.

'If I have to. My lad can drive me. He's waiting in the pickup.'

She moves to help him stand, but he raises a finger to stop her, lurches to his feet, then slowly limps out of the room and down the corridor. You go carefully, she says to his retreating back.

Later that afternoon, the doctor takes a call from the radiographer at the hospital. The farmer has fractured the neck of his right femur. This is so astonishing that the doctor asks whether he could have fallen since she saw him, but the answer is no. The farmer has been walking, and lambing, with a broken hip for a fortnight.

A few weeks after his hip surgery, the doctor makes a home visit to assess his recovery. He mutters about the physiotherapy he's been asked to do. 'A load of nonsense, that is. Told me to use a piece of elastic no bigger than a condom. You seen the size of me?' And, not impolitely, he shows her the door.

A MILE OR SO from the farm, the earth falls away, carved deep by a river. Pastures give way to cliffs and steep gullies knotted with ancient woods and scattered with fragments of lives long past: a maze of old stone walls, tangled paths that lead nowhere, old railway cuttings, heavy with brambles and wild garlic, their only traffic now deer and badgers. As if calibrated not to human time, but to tree time, this valley speaks of the power of nature to reassert itself as people come and go. The handful of villages that lie within it or perch on the slopes above seem like reclaimed land borrowed from a sea of green.

In March 1967, the BBC aired a documentary to coincide with the publication of John Berger's *A Fortunate Man*. It opens with grainy footage of the gaberdine-clad country doctor himself, driving through the valley in his Land Rover. Down a steep wooded lane he goes, then up and over the hump of a bridge, a bank of dark forest ahead, and on through a village, separated from a silvery bend in the river by a thin strip of field. Through the rain-flecked windscreen, not just the contours of the landscape but much of the detail is familiar, uncannily so, more than half a century later: the railings on the bridge, the fence line in the field, the positioning of road signs and tilt of rooftops, the light on the water, the outstretched branches of trees. The world as it was then is the world as it is now, intact, or so it seems, the landscape apparently indifferent to the passage of time.

More than fifty years on, the community remains rural, nominally at least, and the pace of life is still languid, even on a busy day. There are farmers, although fewer than there were, and woodsmen too, although they tend to call themselves 'tree surgeons' these days. Plenty of folk keep a few sheep, or some bees, although not many make their living that way anymore. The valley was never an agricultural heartland, never home to the vast, wealthy farms of the floodplains further north. Many made their crust in the valley quarries, or the small factories of nearby towns, making steam boilers or radiators, fruit cordials or lorry tyres. But home they would come to smallholdings and cider apple orchards that marched downhill to the banks of the river. It was not so long ago, certainly within living memory, that most families would have had a cow out back for milk, maybe a couple of pigs, and all came together at haymaking time or to celebrate the harvest. Only small pockets of that life cling on today.

The modern world has inched its way in, a discreet 4G mast here, a rooftop satellite dish there. Indeed, the bubble of isolation previously so idiomatic to this valley has largely burst. Yes, there are families who've lived here for generations, and remember the maypole every spring, or the winter it snowed so hard, great drifts blew into arches above the narrow lanes, or how a local man who'd fought in the war thereafter washed his hands of humankind and took up residence in a cave beneath the cliff, lichen growing in his beard. However, alongside the old families, there are now incomers, with different stories, jobs elsewhere, children who leave, lives that look out.

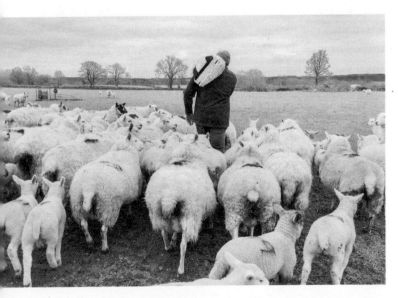

IT'S ONE OF the valley doctor's preferred shortcuts for crossing the village, this path that skirts the graveyard past the grassy tump of a long-gone medieval keep, leading up to the new houses behind the Post Office that's no longer a post office. She's cycling along it when she spots him crossing the damp grass towards the church. She stops and watches him for a moment, as he worries at some creases in his shirt. As a doctor, she's looked after him since he was a boy, although now he is tall and broad, head and shoulders above her.

She calls his name and he turns, walking over to the wall separating path and graveyard. She says how glad she is that he made it and he explains that finals aren't for a few weeks yet, so his tutor gave him the green light to come. 'I couldn't miss it,' he says. She asks about the journey and the hours it must have taken from his university town on the other side of the country. 'I left halls just as it was getting light,' he says. 'Six o'clock coach.' The doctor asks what he's going to play and the young man lifts a carrier bag containing some sheet music. 'It's Bach, and a Parry elegy for the end, as well as the hymns of course.' He tugs again at his shirt. 'Do I look smart enough?' he asks. 'I'm worried it's got crumpled on the bus.' She reassures him and points out that no one can see what you're wearing at the organ anyway. 'I think I'm just a bit nervous,' he says. She mentions that the old lady would love that it was him playing and the young man nods, chews his lip. She has a couple of home visits to do, she says, but she'll be back in time for the service. Then she lifts both hands from the handlebars, fingers crossed. He creaks open the old door of the church, disappears inside.

As the doctor pedals away, her mind tracks back through the young man's story. He had been ten when his father left suddenly, plunging the family, his mother and two siblings, into emotional and financial chaos. That was when they moved here from the city, and over the months that followed, she'd seen a good deal of them at the surgery. Another patient, a woman in her sixties who'd lived all her life on the far side of the village, had recently lost her husband of many years and was struggling with loneliness. So the doctor simply introduced them, the single mother and the new widow, and as she did so, she seeded an idea. Perhaps the boy, who was missing his piano lessons and the instrument they'd had to sell, could practise on the old Chappell upright that stood in the widow's hall?

Over the years, this friendship, so unlikely on the face of it, had blossomed. There were informal piano lessons, impromptu children's teas, birthday presents, all of it a lifeline to the single mother and her children. Later, when the older woman could no longer drive, the roles were reversed: shopping was fetched, her house cleaned, lifts to the surgery given. And today that little boy, now a young man, is to play Bach and Parry on the organ at her funeral.

The NHS might dub this social prescribing or patient participation, a 'neighbourhood care network' perhaps, but the doctor doesn't much care what you call it. There are those among her colleagues who say this is not the job of a GP, that embroiling yourself in the social needs of your patients, at a time when primary care is already overwhelmed, is a recipe for disaster. All the same, the doctor feels a shiver of emotion as she cycles up through the beech woods above the village, thinking of the simple symmetry of help given and help received. She's no dreamer; she knows there's no grand panacea here for a world full of inequity and sorrow. All the same, she's come to recognize these moments of light that flow from knowing your community and knowing your patients, and from connecting the two when you can. It is something a doctor can usefully do with the trust invested in them.

That early impulse with the boy and the piano, more than a decade ago now, was how this idea took shape.

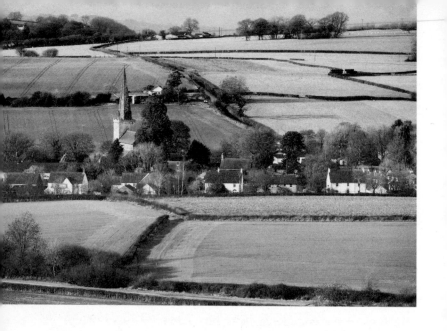

SHE'S EXAMINING the papery soft hip of a woman in her early seventies. It's been aching, the woman says. The doctor rubs her fingers together to warm them, apologizing for her cold hands. 'Gracious, you're right,' says the woman. 'They feel like ice cream.' They laugh at the bane of being a doctor with perennially cold hands. 'We need to knit you some mittens,' says the woman from the consulting couch, as the doctor lifts and flexes her leg, rotating it outward and inward, outward and inward.

She has known this patient for several years, and always found her sunny and garrulous, one of those glass-half-full women who bake sponge cakes for neighbours and give their GP a tin of Quality Street at Christmas. But the doctor has never seen her legs before, she realizes, and one of them tells another story. She touches with a fingertip the milky corrugations of an old scar that runs almost from the woman's knee to her left hip. It gives her leg the look of a crudely stitched rag doll. The doctor asks about it.

'I was ten,' the woman replies. 'I don't think I've ever mentioned it to you, but Dad used to deliver petrol door to door on the other side of the river and sometimes I'd go on his rounds with him before school. This is back when we had quite a few little petrol stations in the valley. He'd work at the pump in the afternoon, but in the morning he'd do a round of people's cars and tractors with a tank on the back of the truck. Where d'you go for petrol now? Into town? We all do. But when I was a girl that was what Dad did and sometimes he'd take me along to open gates and what have you.'

A cloud passes over the woman's face. It makes the doctor stop what she's doing. She covers the woman's lower half with a few paper squares of couch wrap and a murmured 'There.' But she doesn't yet step outside the curtain. She listens.

'So this was one of those mornings when the fog down in the valley is like custard. You drop down the hill into it, don't you, and you can't see your hand in front of you. So there I was, opening a gate for Dad, and this blue Ford Anglia came flying around the bend. The lad driving it swerved so he wouldn't hit Dad's truck and he hit me instead. Pinned me against the fence post in the hedge. He didn't look much older than I was. I can still remember looking down at my leg and seeing this bumper with an L-plate painted on a bit of old box and tied to it with string. Anyway, it broke this big bone here, nasty break, twelve weeks in traction up at the hospital and Mum wasn't allowed to stay with me. You weren't in those days. Then I had a full year in the house, no school, because I couldn't walk. They didn't get you up and about like they do now, so.'

The woman falls quiet. And how, asks the doctor, did that affect you? For a moment, it is as if the woman hasn't heard the question.

'Well, I don't like that valley fog for a start,' she says and stops again. 'D'you know, doctor, no one's ever asked me that, so I've never stopped to think about it. But now I do, well, it blighted my entire life.'

As morning surgery wears on, the doctor tries and fails to shrug off the uncertainty of this encounter, the immensity of it. She finds herself perplexed by time both portioned out in ten-minute appointments and rolling inexorably from child-hood to old age. For the rest of the day, the doctor herself feels wreathed in river mist, where nothing is quite as it seems.

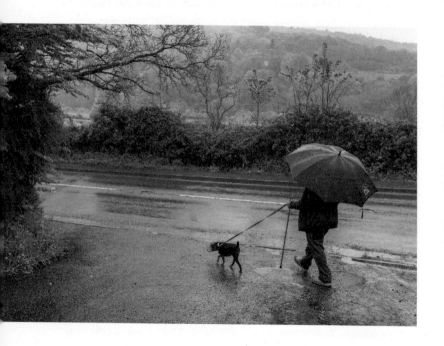

SHE WAS SITTING on his garden wall, the doctor, when he got back.

He had woken not long after five that Saturday morning, just as the rising sunlight touched the rooftops of the houses on the far side of the valley. Above the cacophony of a spring dawn, and the bellowing of a solitary ram in the field below, he could hear the blood roaring in his ears. That was what woke him, that or a strange pressure in his chest, as if an unseen hand had got hold of last night's chicken dinner and was wrenching at it inside him. His wife had stirred and he'd told her he felt 'bloody awful'. She had eyed him carefully, but he'd said, 'No, stop it, I'm fine', taken an aspirin and gone back to sleep. Come breakfast time, his wife's protests that he should get to the hospital, if only as a precaution, had been batted away. 'Nah, I'm alright', and off he'd gone to replace a couple of slates on a roof in the next village and collect some bales. It was when he returned that he found the doctor, in her weekend civvies, jeans and walking boots, sitting on the stone wall outside the cottage. She often walked her dogs up through the woods that rose between their two houses. They'd been neighbours for nigh-on twenty years and it wasn't unusual for her to stop and chat. But there were no dogs with her today. Instead, he spied a certain resolve in her face as she smiled when his van pulled in.

'I've been waiting for you,' she said.

He greeted her by her first name. They had never bothered with the 'Doctor' honorific. He'd always considered them friends, although, like pretty much everyone around here, she was also his doctor and had seen him through a thing or two over the years. 'Absolutely bloody perfectly straight as a die' is how he liked to describe her, although he was glad never to have had to see her for any 'boy problems, shall we say?' This would always make him laugh and the doctor roll her eyes, but this wasn't a day for jokes.

'Helen came over,' she said. 'Says you're not feeling so good. I was out walking, so she's been driving round the woods looking for me.'

He mumbled a few words about indigestion, but she challenged him. 'Helen always says you could eat a vindaloo and a box of rusty nails and you'd not feel a thing. You look awful.'

He met her eye, murmuring something about the bales he wanted to unload, but the clamminess of his brow gave him away. 'Come on.' Her voice was low, stern. 'You know and Helen knows and I know you've had chest pains.' She asked if the pain was still there and he tipped a hand back and forth, saying that he'd been planning to see her at the surgery on Monday if he didn't feel better. Glancing at her watch, she asked when they had started, and what it felt like. He told her, describing the sensation of pressure, a heaviness or a squeezing at the very top of his belly.

'That sounds horrible for you. OK, so what we need you to do now is to get in the car with Helen and go straight to A&E. She's already told me you don't want to, but she's right, you must. We need to find out what's going on, don't we, and they've got all the kit up there to do that. So she's coming out now. There she is.' She nodded to the face that had just appeared at the kitchen window. 'It could take an ambulance an hour to get here, so I think it's a better idea to leave now. Helen's going to drive and you'll be there in forty minutes.'

He started to protest. He'd got things to do. He was probably OK.

'This is not about "probably".' She used his name, slowed her voice. 'This is about us doing what we need to do. And if we don't, it's asking for trouble. You know I wouldn't say that if I didn't mean it. You know I'm not one to make a fuss. Have I ever lied to you?'

Like a chastened schoolboy, he shook his head.

'No. So it's time to go.' Her voice softened. 'There. Well done. You're a star. They'll sort you out. They know what they're doing up there. Helen will keep me posted.'

As the car pulled out, she waved them off with a bright smile and a thumbs up, then turned on her heels and disappeared into the thick green of the path below. At the hospital, they told him he'd had a heart attack, but stabilized him, and a week later, he was discharged. Over the months that followed, again and again he would replay that Saturday morning in his mind, as a succession of hypotheticals. 'I mean, I wouldn't have gone, would I? I would have carried on working and had a bigger attack very shortly, wouldn't I? But she gave me a rollicking and it probably saved my life, didn't it?'

At those moments, an almost physical understanding of his neighbour's job would blaze in his mind, that her whole life was made up of questions like this, questions for which you might never know the answer. He'd follow her to the ends of the earth now.

NOT EVERYONE FEELS like this about the doctor. Some weeks earlier, a patient had attended the surgery with, as she made abundantly clear, the utmost reluctance. A gaunt, well-tailored woman in her sixties, she'd been registered for several years, but had never darkened the doctor's door until today. She said there was no need to sit down, nor indeed to outline the nature of her complaint. She would just, if doctor would oblige, like some antibiotics.

'I don't like doctors,' the woman said.

Why not? asked the doctor. Have you had a difficult experience?

The woman ignored the second question, but answered the first with what appeared to be a modicum of relish. 'It is,' she said, 'because they are incompetent, mendacious and venal. The antibiotics please.'

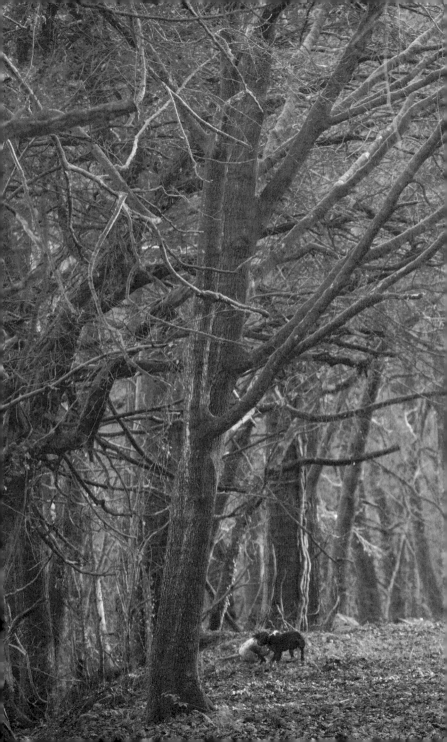

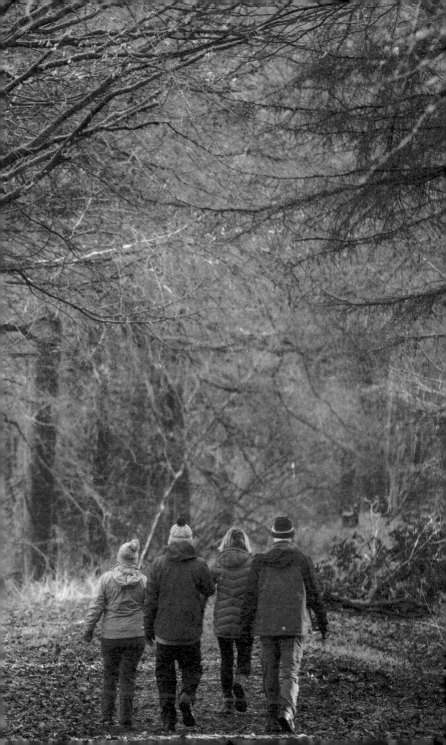

OF THE NEARLY five thousand patients registered with the practice, there are many the valley doctor won't see from one year to the next. They don't need her; they are busy living. Indeed, the arc of a life is reflected in who appears in the consulting room, and when. During the first two or three years of life, she frequently sees her infant patients with childhood coughs and colds. Thereafter, healthy children largely disappear from her appointment list, with girls returning briefly during puberty with spots or period pain, and later for contraception. Among younger female patients, birth control continues to be a theme, followed in due course by its opposite, as many of them reappear with pregnancies and babies, before vanishing again until menopause. In the case of male patients, it's common for a general practitioner to lose them in mid-childhood, when small boys have more or less worked out how to keep themselves in one piece, and not see them again until several decades later. Then, finally, the inevitable: as the human body awakens to its own finitude, patients, both male and female, reacquaint themselves with the doctor's consulting room and, over the autumnal years of life, grow to rely upon the interventions and the reassurance they find there. Clearly, there are manifold exceptions at every stage, wild-card pathologies, untimely storms of body or mind, and these too lie within the doctor's purview. And yet no two patients, no two people, are ever the same. Pay attention to this, above all, and it will make you not just a nicer doctor, but a better doctor. Of that she is certain.

For there extends behind every encounter the doctor has, on every day of her working life, not just a medical history but also a personal history, a winding corridor of experience and emotion, the patient's whole life. In any given consultation, she is afforded but a fragment, a scintilla of that history. It is one of the joys of being a long-serving family doctor in a community like this, that she has both time and opportunity to piece the fragments together, over years and across families and generations. She was taught, and she strives to remember, that this is what general practice is all about, talking to people, listening to their stories, every bit as much as it's about clinical examination. On days when the administrative paperwork piles high, these stories are what keeps her going. They are the raw material of her relationship with each patient and a source of endless complexity and fascination. That's why the doctor keeps a thick hardback notebook in which she jots a line or two about the most interesting case of each day, the one that makes her wonder about people, marvel at them or despair. She sometimes says to fellow bookworms (who she knows will find the analogy resonant) that her job is like picking your way through some wonderful library with extraordinary tales on every shelf. Reduce any one of your patients to their affliction, the tumorous breast, incompetent heart valve or lazy pancreas, and it's akin to regarding a book as nothing more than paper and ink.

Besides, she knows that the corridor of experience and emotion, the patient's story, doesn't stop here. It extends in the other direction too, stretching darkly into the future, and for that she holds a degree of responsibility.

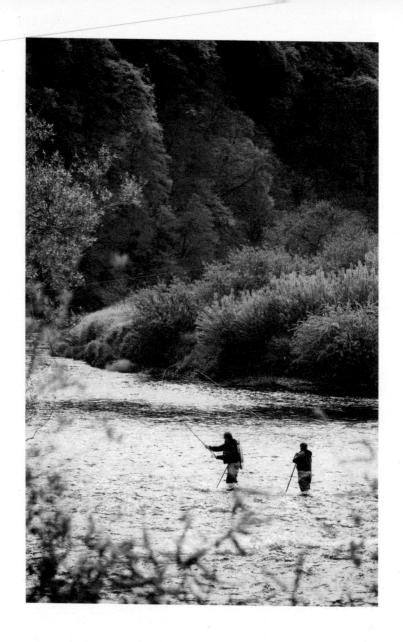

THE DISTRICT NURSE is just finishing up when the doctor arrives to review the man's pain medication. So she waits in the hall, beneath a framed and now-yellowing school photograph of a young man with all his life ahead of him. The year it was taken, 1996, is embossed in gold on the brown cardboard mount. The patient's wife steps out of the kitchen with a cup of tea, the steam of it rising in the sunshine that pours through the etched glass above the front door.

'Sorry, doctor, kettle was whistling. She's still in there, the nurse. Won't be long, I don't think. Cup of tea?'

The doctor declines. She never confuses home visits with tea breaks, but she's happy to talk and asks about the patient, how he's been.

'He's alright.' The woman pauses, knowing this is not strictly true. 'Yes, but he is, he's alright. The nights are hard, but that's how it is.'

The doctor can see the tiredness in the woman's eyes. She asks how she is coping.

'Oh, I'm not too bad. I'm managing. You know us. We find our little ways to keep each other smiling. Always have. Even after Tom.' She nods towards the photo on the wall and there's a short pause. 'But we're forty-two years wed, you know, and . . . well, it helps.'

At that moment, the living-room door flies open and the district nurse bustles out.

'Sorry to keep you, doctor. One of us will be back and see him tomorrow late morning.' She turns to the man's wife. 'SO HE'S ALL SORTED, PET.' She enunciates each word, *fortissimo*. 'YOU GOT THAT? HE'S ALL SORTED, SO DON'T YOU WORRY, YOU'RE DOING GRAND. WE'LL BE ALONG AND SEE YOU TOMORROW AND YOU HAVE THE NUMBER TO CALL IF THERE'S ANY PROBLEM, ALRIGHTY?'

33

'I've got the number in the kitchen, thank you,' says the dying man's wife, the ghost of a smile in her eyes.

The minute the front door closes behind the district nurse, a crackle of hoarse laughter can be heard from the hospital bed that's been wheeled in front of the fireplace in the living room.

'Last week, when she started, that new nurse, *he*, the cheeky bugger' – the woman nods towards the thin, ashy figure in the bed next door – 'he thought it would be funny to tell her his wife was very deaf and also a bit slow. I haven't had the heart to set her right. Anyway, you go on in. He's waiting for you.'

The joke works. That split second of private dread that periodically assails the doctor on the threshold of a dying man or woman dissolves. She steps through, brisk and bright, into the room.

WHEN THE LARCHES in the grove at the top of the beacon shed in November, their amber needles fill the air like falling snow. They settle on the doctor's gloved hands and the sleeves of her jacket as she cycles towards evening surgery on the other side of the valley. The track through this woodland begins not far from one surgery and leads up and over a heath, before dropping sharply to the valley floor. There, a cast-iron bridge spans the river and a steep climb awaits through oaks and ancient chestnuts to the village and the other surgery above. The journey takes the doctor twenty-seven minutes.

Whenever she describes this commute to colleagues at medical conferences or faculty meetings, she's conscious that it sounds almost parodically old-world, especially to urban doctors. So she always points out that hers is a state-of-the-art e-bike – the hills would be unconscionable otherwise – and that it's part of trying to make hers a greener practice, with minimal car use for home visits or between sites. It also makes it easier when citing the mental and physical health benefits of exercise to patients if she isn't entirely sedentary herself; that, and the fact that without this daily hour out of doors she would surely go mad. For, although this is not something the doctor cares to mention often, these rides are when the weight of the job comes off her, blowing away like larch needles as she cycles downhill.

The doctor chooses not to dwell on the dark side of her work. Quite the reverse, she casts herself, and not just to others, as the most fortunate of women. Here she is, in the loveliest valley in the world, with a job she adores, one that does palpable good in her community, stimulates her intellect and more than pays the bills, all of it just a mile or two on foot or bike from the pretty stone house where, at the end of every day, her husband and two children are waiting.

Nevertheless, it is impossible to forget, dangerous to forget, what this job can do to you. The doctor before last in this practice – yes, John Berger's 'Fortunate Man', John Sassall – took his own life in 1982, just weeks after retirement. The community he had served for thirty-five years was traumatized by his death. Some days, this lingers in the doctor's mind as the most vivid of warnings.

On such days, the darkness crowds in. She recollects, for instance, that she's never met a GP who couldn't tell you the name, age and circumstances of every suicide they've ever had to deal with; she certainly can. Or she recalls her humiliation at the funeral of a young cancer patient, where she found herself, the local doctor, for God's sake, in tears at the back of the church. She acknowledges the oppressive, sleep-disrupting difficulty of intervening, or not intervening, in an abusive marriage between a well-heeled lawyer and his vulnerable wife, who comes to the surgery with headaches and weeps silently. She shudders at how a tiny error in the labelling of a blood test saw her driving thirty miles to a city laboratory between morning and evening surgeries, afraid that a pregnant patient, who'd spent years trying to have a baby, would miscarry.

Most of the time, at least, these things go unsaid, and an hour speeding through dappled woods is part of this doctor's survival strategy.

A FEW YEARS BACK, she was moved to contemplate the ripples that fan out from any human undoing like that of John Sassall, often in inscrutable ways.

It was morning surgery and the front desk rang to say an elderly man was waiting for her by reception. His name was familiar. He had lived these last forty years in the same butter-yellow cottage at the end of the steep lane beyond the old well at the edge of the village. Yet she could not recall his ever having made an appointment to see her, in all the time she'd been the doctor here. She checked the notes. Nothing on the computer. So she stepped into the back office and leafed through the paper files that preceded the arrival, somewhat late, of the white heat of technology to this rural practice. Sure enough, his last appointment had been in 1982, when he was in his early forties.

As is her habit, the doctor walked up the corridor to fetch the elderly man from the waiting room. She finds this brief prelude secures her a few valuable seconds to extend an assessment, to gauge the patient's mood, their expression and complexion, how they move, how they breathe. Yet on this occasion, her overriding impression was of nothing so much as the patient's reticence, as if he were not at all sure that this visit to the doctor was wise.

Once seated in the consulting room, his doubt had seemed to linger. She attempted to break the ice by saying how nice it was to meet him properly and mentioned that it was thirty-three years since his last appointment.

'Yeah, well,' he said, 'the last doctor I saw was Dr Sassall, mind, and he shot himself soon after, so . . .'

The old man didn't finish his sentence. A fallow silence followed; then the consultation began.

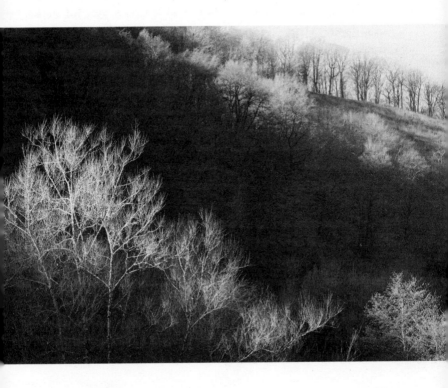

AT THE CREST of the valley, above the village through which Dr Sassall drives in the 1967 film, there stands a fine Victorian country house, now repurposed as a residential nursing home. It overlooks a stretch of the river that runs poker straight for over half a mile, the opposing bank a wall of uninterrupted woodland, dark and lush. Nearby is a set of waterfalls that roll through a deep ravine from the top of the valley to its floor. The roar of the water in the winter months can be heard from the nursing-home steps. The village too tumbles down the steep slope below. It has an almost alpine appearance when viewed from the fields upstream, each house neatly pressed above another into the forest soil, as if to stop them plummeting downhill. The people whose cottages cling to the upper portions of the village describe their neighbours below as living 'downstairs'. Indeed the hillside is criss-crossed with a network of old stone steps laid two centuries ago onto ancient donkey tracks when the village was a hub for river trade. The grand house, now the nursing home at the top of the hill, was built by an affluent family of river barge operators, who ran great teams of harnessed men to haul the barges upstream by rope.

The labour of these men sometimes flashes across the doctor's mind as she too labours on her bike up the spindly lane at the back of the village. Much loathed today by delivery drivers, it is oppressively narrow and steep, but every Monday fifty or so of her most complex patients are waiting for her in the nursing home at the top. Such a wealth of life within those walls, so many ethical conundrums to unravel, she has grown to love this place, its winding corridors and its surprises.

Before tackling the climb, the doctor often makes a pit stop at the village stores at the bottom of the hill for a square of lardy cake (baked on Thursdays), or something from one of the large jars behind the counter. The doctor is fond of sweets. It's a happy day when she remembers she has half a paper bag of lemon bonbons tucked deep in her doctor's case. She sometimes says that her plan for old age is to live on sweets and audiobooks. Not that that day seems near. Even in early middle age, she exudes the energy of a woman half her years. 'How does she fit it all in?' people murmur, as she is seen strapping canoes to the roof of her car before morning surgery, or jogging in the woods with a head torch when most people have finished their dinner and are just putting the bins out before bed. Perhaps the sweets help. In any event, this respect for the life-affirming properties of confectionery may account for the doctor's affinity with the patient she is seeing this morning.

The old lady, well into her nineties, is lying in the foetal position, encased by a womb of bolsters and pillows that the nursing-home staff have propped around her. Her birdlike frame – she weighs no more than forty kilos – is dwarfed by the hospital bed where she has lain for the better part of a decade. It was eight years ago now that the doctor, the head nurse and the lady's devoted family decided that physiotherapy was achieving nothing and was simply too distressing for her. At this point, her children, pensioners in their own right, were told that she was to be placed on the palliative register, a list of the doctor's patients for whom it would be unsurprising if death came within the next six months.

It's no accident that this criterion lacks a certain precision. Caring for patients in the final months of life has long been bread-and-butter work for family physicians. However, in recent decades its profile in health policy has risen, as the ageing population grows and people are increasingly living longer with serious health conditions. The palliative care register, implemented in 2006, was part of a move to encourage GPs to get to grips with this growing constituency teetering close to the precipice of life. The motivation was a good one: it was about ensuring the best end-of-life care. Yet any GP will tell you that it remains notoriously difficult to define when living becomes dying, with no clear consensus upon where to confect a boundary. Does it come one year out, six months out, six weeks out, six days, six hours, six minutes, six seconds? Because of course, at a materialist level, it doesn't; not until death itself.

Besides, the doctor herself has grown accustomed to the uncertainty. She sees the value of the protocol, but has learned over the years not to try and tidy up the untidyable. Recognizing the end of life with certain pathologies, such as cancer, has become easier, but there are others, heart failure or chronic respiratory disease, which remain as tricky to second-guess as ever. And at the top of this enigmatic heap, you find frail old ladies, who have a habit of astonishing their doctors with their tenacious hold on life.

So here, eight years on, the old lady remains in her nursing-home bed, immobile and not much given to interaction anymore, but with an impressive heap of sweets on her bedside table: Rolos, Maltesers, Jelly Babies. The doctor has no idea how she accesses them. Reaching up there is out of the question. Yet every week there are different packets and tubes of sugary loveliness, half-finished, next to the bed. She must, the doctor decides, prompt her carers to pop one into her mouth. Indeed, in spite of her miniature form, the notes at the bottom of her bed indicate that she eats three meals a day, apparently with gusto. Everyone agrees she is a miracle of survival.

When the doctor makes her weekly ward round, the old lady's children often ask her to check their mother's chest, which is always clear – but not today. When she tucks the stethoscope inside the brushed cotton of the old lady's nightgown, she can hear a sound like a gust of wind hitting a microphone. She listens again to be sure, then she crouches down by the bed so that her face is level with the patient's and she explains that there seems to be a chest infection.

'What?' the old lady exclaims, immediately alert. 'A chest infection? Damned chest! How has this happened?'

Her animation is as surprising as it is palpable.

'Will that see me off?' she asks. 'Dear God, then what are we going to do about it, doctor?'

For a second, the doctor and the nurse in attendance exchange a glance of amazement. The old lady hasn't been this lively in years, but now appears urgently galvanized by the idea that the infection might do her harm. The doctor explains that a course of antibiotics would be the next logical step.

'Well, absolutely. Let's be getting rid of the damn thing.'

This fierce will to live burns quietly under winceyette night-gowns and checked pyjamas everywhere, often in the most unexpected places. The doctor knows this. It is one of the great privileges of her work that she is afforded glimpses of it, like this one. The antibiotics work, the infection passes and the old lady is still enjoying her sweets six months later.

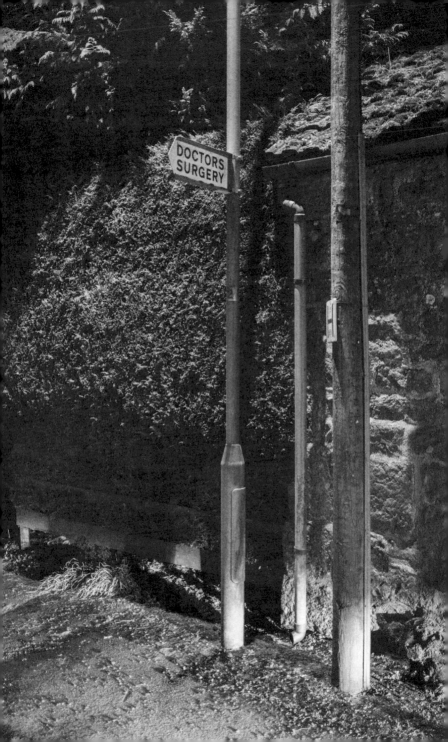

THE VOLUME OF BLOOD was terrifying.

The woman had called the surgery earlier in the day. She was twenty-three weeks pregnant and concerned that she'd barely felt her baby move for a day or more. Not the usual sharp kick in the ribs, she told the receptionist, nor that shove to the bladder that had made her heart sing these last few weeks. This was her fifth pregnancy. All four previous pregnancies had ended in miscarriage, two in the second trimester. The doctor knew the woman well and had seen her in the surgery after the latter two miscarriages. Each time, there had been a name for the baby and an imagined future; each loss had been devastating, with a payload of guilt and a deep sadness that she told the doctor she felt would never go away. The last time, the woman had said how much she had come to hate the word 'miscarriage', with all its overtones of badness and wrongness. She would never use the word again, she said, just 'I lost him' or 'I lost her', although this too made her weep at her careless body.

The doctor had remembered this when the receptionist mentioned her call, and immediately fitted the woman in at evening surgery, hopeful that she would find the baby's heartbeat and set her mind at rest. They'd met in the village only a few weeks before and gushed joyfully together about how well this pregnancy was going, how she'd never got this far before, how happy, hopeful and scared she felt.

Now the woman lay back on the consulting couch, slipping an oversized Minnie Mouse T-shirt above the pale dome of her abdomen.

'Yesterday, I felt a bit of fluttering,' she said, 'but now, nothing at all.' She instinctively placed both palms either side of her bump, as if divining for water.

The doctor made some soothing small talk as she turned to fetch the foetal Doppler from a drawer, but suddenly she heard the woman catch her breath.

'Oh no. I think I'm bleeding.'

The doctor turned back to see a pool of bright red blood gathering beneath the woman's hips, soaking through her leggings onto the white paper of the couch and now beginning to drip onto the floor.

'Oh God,' the woman whispered.

A spike of adrenaline and now the doctor did what she always does when she's afraid. She slowed down, checking her movements and her voice to a deliberate calm, as if proceeding underwater. She took an incontinence pad from the cupboard in the corridor, slid it under the woman's hips and called 999 from the phone on the desk.

An antepartum haemorrhage on this scale is a possible sign that the placenta, fed by a mass of blood vessels, has lifted away from the wall of the uterus. Placental abruption, as it is called, can be dangerous for the baby, and, with bleeding as heavy as this, also dangerous for the mother.

The doctor checked the woman's blood pressure, explaining that she was going to give her some fluids. Just a little boost, keep it all stable. *Cannula in. Saline up. Jesus, the blood.* In the far recesses of the doctor's mind, four questions circled each other, like a mobile over an infant's cot. *Is the baby going to die? Is the baby already dead? Is the woman going to bleed out right here? Is she going to die because I have somehow failed?*

A ragged sob came from the couch. 'I've tried so hard to do everything right,' the woman said. 'I've been so careful. I'm just trying to think what I might have . . .'

The doctor explained that the drip was now replacing some of the lost fluid, so not to worry. Even a little blood looks like a lot, you know.

'I did go to a Zumba class. D'you think that . . .'

Just keep calm. Think what it's like, the doctor said, if you spill a pint of milk on the kitchen floor. It's only a pint, but it looks like a gallon, and remember you've got lots of pints.

'Yes, but still, this isn't like a period or anything. It's like a tap.'

The woman was right, but the doctor didn't say so, just continued murmuring reassurances. She always endeavours to be as honest as possible with her patients. It's a promise she makes several times a week: 'I'll always be straight with you.' She's learned over the years, with cancers and other mortal news, that candour is the best policy; say the scary word, puncture the taboo, and you and the patient can begin to work together on what to do next. But were she to say to this young woman in the Minnie Mouse T-shirt, 'It is my belief that the baby is already dead and your life is in the balance', it would not help in any way. Keeping the woman calm was a medical necessity, and candour could wait.

So the ambulance is on its way, the doctor said, keeping her voice light. Might take a little while, she said, but not too long to wait now.

'And the roads,' said the woman, 'it's all lanes, isn't it, the last six or seven miles?' Her terror was like a solid thing in the room.

Let's have another one of those, said the doctor cosily, replacing the blood-drenched pad with a fresh one. Drawing as little attention to it as possible, she had done this three or four times in twenty minutes.

'My baby, my baby,' murmured the woman, tears streaking down into her hair. 'Can you listen for a heartbeat?'

The doctor had been dreading this question. She delayed, explaining that a heartbeat wouldn't necessarily change anything. The ambulance would be here any minute. If we hear the baby, that's wonderful, she said, but it doesn't necessarily mean that everything is alright, not with this bleeding. But the truth was the doctor didn't think they were going to hear the baby. She thought what they'd hear was silence.

'Please,' the woman said.

And if we don't hear anything, the doctor went on, then we'll both be upset and it'll make things harder for you.

'I just need to know,' said the woman.

Round and round this conversation went.

'Please, please, please, I just need to know.'

So, with nowhere to go, the doctor took the Doppler, smeared some gel on the woman's firm belly and together they listened for the 'shh-shh-shh-shh' of a tiny heart beating.

My God, said the doctor, you were right. You knew. There we go.

'Shh-shh-shh-shh-shh-shh . . .'

It's the best sound in the whole wide world, isn't it, said the doctor. Let's hold on to that, shall we? Let's hold on to that and just hope as hard as we can. And for a moment, they were not doctor and patient, just two women together, terrified and hopeful.

The ambulance arrived and as the woman was stretchered away, the doctor called out. She'd phone Dave, yes, she'd got his number, she'd get him to go straight there. 'I'll be thinking about you all the time,' the doctor said.

By some benign twist of nature, all was well, and when the doctor went to visit them three months later, their house was a riot of pink balloons and banners. Nearly a decade on, the woman, now in her forties, and her daughter are still the doctor's patients. They never speak about that day. She doubts the woman dwells on it much, but the doctor cannot see the girl without a lump in her throat and a thought for how fragile the line between joy and despair.

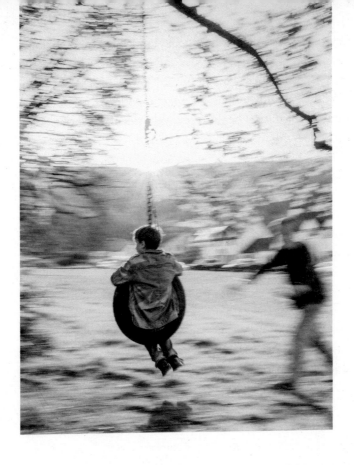

As THE SUN SINKS in the valley and the shadows rise, as if from the waters of the river itself, the people who live here go about their business. An elderly man crouches on his garden step, brushing his dog's grinning teeth with a small toothbrush. A teenager, bare to the waist, LA hip-hop blaring, practises kick-flips on his skateboard in a fluorescent-lit garage. A woman in office clothes heaves bags of shopping from the boot of her car onto the mossy flagstones by her back door. A couple walking hand in hand stop on a rusty footbridge and they kiss. A man in painter's overalls swirls his brushes in turps by a kitchen sink overlooking the darkening forest, and hums a thread of melody. A baby drifts off to sleep, wrapped tight in a woven blanket, the sound of wood pigeons cooing outside her window. And at the surgery, their doctor bumps her bike over the back step, turns off the light inside and begins the lovely ride towards home.

II

It was no bigger than the palm of her hand, a smooth oval of perfection, like a river pebble in the early evening sunshine.

She was treading in divots after school in the field where the foals were grazing. It was a pleasant, meditative way to end the day, tucking her plimsoll toe under each clod of turf turned by the mares' hooves, flipping it over and pressing the ground back to a smooth, satisfying green. She and her parents had moved some months earlier from the gorse-clad hills further west to this verdant paddock. Here they'd embarked upon the latest of a succession of rural enterprises, this time breeding racehorses. A new home meant yet another new school, the eighth of an itinerant childhood, so here she was, halfway through a lonely first year at a nearby sixth-form college. Yet there was something about her, a collision of innate optimism with a kind of conscientious attention to the present, that meant even difficult times did not preclude moments of euphoric insight. She was always like that, and still is.

So there it was, tucked into a dimple within the lush green of the field: a leveret, perfectly still, its eyes wide, its long ears flattened against its back, almost as if it were carved in stone.

She strode towards it, thinking it was a divot. When she realized it was not a clump of earth, but a tiny new life, she wrestled briefly with an urge to scoop it up and take it home. There had been various poorly creatures over the years to whom she had offered sanctuary. The most beloved was Noddy, the pet goose, hatched in her bedroom from an abandoned egg. Noddy grew to be a magnificent fowl that would sit and honk from the little girl's lap, only to be stolen by some heartless wretch just before Christmas. But this evening in the field, she thought better of a heroic rescue and retreated to watch at a distance. Sure enough, the mother hare soon loped into view. Long limbed and eared, she tended to her baby for some minutes, before finally darting off and disappearing into a hedge, leaving the teenage girl in a state of quiet bliss.

The knowledge that nature can offer up such moments of stillness and consolation has never left her. More than three decades on, she can still recall in detail that leveret and its mother. The encounter felt meaningful, a spark of wonder at the living world that has been renewed many times over the years. Such moments of magic, a constellation of small epiphanies, sit like pins on the map of her life, a source of contentment and affirmation to this day.

These little flashes of inspiration, when life seems to pivot, are often a feature of the late teens. It's almost as if nature requires a confluence of high emotion, impulsivity and clarity in order to nudge us over the brink from childhood into the adult world. For her, the not-yet-doctor, this was one of three such moments in as many months, when heart and head seemed to align, passion and intellect join forces. Another came, in classic teenage fashion, with her discovery of a song that touched her to the core with its plea for connection and communication. Even today, she still listens to Simon & Garfunkel's 'The Sound of Silence' on her headphones as she cycles through the valley, or rolls the song through her mind, mantra-like, in moments of tension. Bleak though the sentiment, it soothes her. However, the most significant revelation of those months towards the end of her childhood came with the reading of a book.

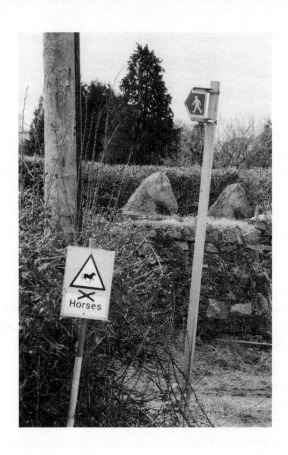

NEITHER OF HER PARENTS had gone to university. Her mother, bright and rebellious, had been just sixteen when she'd met her future husband at the local riding stables in a rural backwater. Love at first sight led to bouts of truancy and her provincial English grammar school suggested she might as well leave there and then. This had so irritated the young woman that she'd worked hard and left school that summer with nine O levels. The following year, at seventeen, her baby daughter was born, with similar grit and intelligence, it seems. Their only child, she grew up bookish and determined not to be pigeonholed, as happy in gumboots hefting bales as she was in the school library, her nose in a novel.

Although her family was proudly working class, there were always horses around and for the first fourteen years of her life, the girl was never planning to be anything other than a jockey. Even now in the study at home, where she works late into the evening, writing referral letters or reading medical papers, there is a photograph of her eleven-year-old self plunging into the waters of a lake astride a raven-black horse, her skull cap silk stitched by her mother with yellow ribbon stripes. Through several house-moves and changes of school, it was her love of horses that provided something like continuity. There would be days at the races with her father, a committed gambler and eternal optimist, ever hopeful that tomorrow would be their lucky day. Money came and went. One day it was steak for dinner, the next baked beans. But before long, there she'd be again, following him in his trainer's hat through a racecourse crowd, watching the pockets of his waxed jacket at his strict instruction, lest a light-fingered punter relieve him of the fistful of twenties won on some propitious thoroughbred. It was from her father that she says her optimism comes.

She was a busy little girl, and would routinely fall out with her best friend, who walked too slowly even if she carried the friend's bags to speed things up. There was simply too much to do to waste time dawdling. From the age of ten or so, she kept a diary in which the events of each day were ordered and contained, plans rehearsed, the future mapped. It was here that a half-formed idea of studying medicine first appeared some-time around her fourteenth birthday. Her school grades were certainly good enough, but the inspiration came in part from a dynamic med student cousin of hers, who used to visit in his bug-eyed Sprite and would take her for a spin. To the mild bafflement of her parents, she had promptly switched mid-term

from humanities and languages to a full se\
primary school nickname of 'Mad-Horse' ga\
one, not entirely kind: 'Please-Miss'. By sixt.\
she was more or less fixed on medical school,\
the application process was hard, even back thei.\
of work experience was considered a good bet. She\
the October half term of lower sixth shadowing her c ..t ramily
doctor in a nearby market town. And so came to pass the third
and most important epiphany of that year of being seventeen.

The GP with whom she spent the week was very funny in
a dry, cynical sort of way, but also passionate about general
practice, keen to point out that this was the only branch of
medical practice that defines its work in terms of relationships.
To illustrate the point, he recommended an old book about a
rural doctor in the 1960s that she really must read. He turned
the surgery shelves upside down to search for his copy, but it
couldn't be found, so she left that Friday afternoon with just
the title and author scrawled on a scrap of paper: *A Fortunate
Man* by John Berger. They didn't have it in the town library,
so she ordered it up from the county stacks. A few weeks
later it arrived, a cellophane-wrapped hardback with thick-
ened brownish pages, furry at the edge, and that unmistakable
library book smell. The book was a few years older than she
was, she noticed, and clearly well thumbed, with two decades'
worth of stamps on the flyleaf.

She began reading on the bus home and devoured *A Fortunate Man* in two days, curled up on a beanbag below the
skylight window in her attic bedroom. As soon as she finished
it, she turned to the beginning and started again.

She had no idea where the book was set – it didn't seem to
matter – but poring over this account of what it meant to be
a doctor sealed something in her young mind. At first read,
she was drawn to the drama, not least of the opening scene in

meet the country doctor in crisis mode attending man pinned by a fallen tree. It felt almost as if this were some grown-up version of the pony adventure stories of her childhood, the plucky girl who saves the day now transposed as the steadfast doctor who fights for the woodsman's mangled leg. However, at second read, a measure of the breadth and psychological complexity of the doctor's work began to sink in. There was something beguiling in this dual role of clinical expert and compassionate witness to people's stories and their struggles over time. It was a book about relationships and relationships matter when you're an only child who's moved schools seven times. Here was a glimpse of the stability, continuity and connection that she so craved, but without, as she saw it, sacrificing skill, intellect, aspiration.

She returned *A Fortunate Man* to the library and went straight to the second-hand bookshop in a neighbouring town to buy her own copy. More than thirty years later, it still sits, between a textbook on symptom management in advanced cancer and the British National Formulary for Children, on the shelf above the desk in her consulting room.

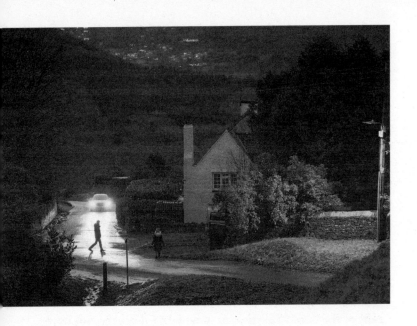

THE DOCTOR CAST BY John Berger as 'Dr John Sassall' died in 1982, six years before his seventeen-year-old would-be successor, two counties away, first read about his life. Although she didn't know it then, the figure of Sassall already enjoyed a quasi-mythic status within medical literature, widely regarded as a high-water mark for all that the doctor–patient relationship could encompass. *A Fortunate Man* was, and to an extent still is, considered a definitive account of the ideals that underlie general practice. It was not at all unusual for doctors to recommend the book as required reading for trainee medics or eager sixth-formers applying for medical school. Yet, long before its tragic postscript, *A Fortunate Man* was already a melancholy book, perhaps because it didn't flinch from the reality of what medicine can and cannot achieve in ameliorating the human condition, perhaps because it absorbed a little of the despair that intermittently engulfed its protagonist. From the moment

Berger's ink dried and Mohr's photographs swam into focus in their darkroom trays, the book was tinged with loss. Indeed, over the years, as healthcare has modernized (and modernized again), the devoted, complex, tireless Dr Sassall has become the conduit of a certain nostalgia for the days when long-term relationships were the heart of general practice, his name a byword for the profound value of continuity of care.

It is curious, then, that this deathless fame in the world of medical letters, and the hushed reverence accorded to Sassall both in the UK and overseas, is not much replicated today in the valley where he lived and worked. The stories that linger here seem earthier somehow, more knotty in their contradictions – that is, if they are remembered at all.

With the notable exception of the lead doctor herself, nobody working in Sassall's old practice, when I first made contact, had heard of the book: not the part-time salaried doctor, not in the back office or among the small team of nurses and healthcare assistants. One of the surgery's pharmacy dispensers, now in her forties, has lived here all her life and she certainly remembers queuing up with her brother, aged five or six, outside the narrow building that used to be Sassall's surgery. She can recall the doctor looking sternly at her, painfully probing the glands beneath her jawline – *'Does that hurt? No? You're fine. There's nothing wrong with you.'* – and bundling the two children back out into the damp green lane; but of the book, she knew nothing. Most people around here know that one of the Spice Girls used to live in a house on the other side of the river, and that a couple of television presenters reside in lovely old farmhouses in the woods nearby, but of the 'fortunate man', only shreds of recollection remain. The world moves on, its values shift, and even the most dedicated servants of the community recede in the collective memory, like old millstones forgotten in the woods, now overgrown with moss and ivy.

There are, however, a handful who do remember 'Dr John', as they call him, and are happy to share their reminiscences. His surviving son was in the latter stages of terminal cancer when we talked early in 2021. He spoke of how proud he was 'of the old man', in spite of what was clearly a complicated relationship. 'I wish I could talk to him again,' he said. 'To be honest, he haunts me to death, not just because of the respect in which he was held by the community, but also because of the book.'

His father had arrived in the valley to deep snow during the brutally cold January of 1947, eighteen months before the NHS was established. Fresh from a spell as a navy surgeon, this was to be his first and only medical practice, and the son spoke of how in the autumn of the following year, his father had written a polite, personal letter to each of his patients telling them, *You are now part of the National Health Service, so you don't need to pay me anymore, thank you very much.* He described how 'totally, totally central' to his father's identity being the doctor in this community was, and how over the thirty-five years he worked here, he had fashioned the practice in his own maverick image. 'You'd not be able to do this nowadays, but he lived his life as a doctor as he wanted to live it.' Although the home visit was still a staple of general practice at that time, Dr John favoured seeing his patients at the one-room surgery, with all his instruments and medications to hand. He procured a second-hand VW camper van, which he would send about the valley to collect patients and bring them up to his small consulting room, appointed with faded domestic furniture. 'He installed a direct line up to the surgery from our house,' said his son, 'so people were told, "When you get there, ring down on the landline from the waiting room and I'll be up with you in five minutes." That was the technology of the day, his Land Rover, the VW and a phone.'

Grateful patients in those early years of the NHS often struggled to comprehend the boon of healthcare free at the point of delivery. One patient, the owner of a nearby timber mill, refloored the doctor's family home in maple as a mark of his gratitude; another, whose dying wife had been cared for by Dr John, bought the surgery one of the first electrocardiogram machines to be installed in a rural practice anywhere in the country. 'I was the initial guinea pig on that ECG machine,' the son said.

Berger's book may have haunted Dr John's son, but among most who live here today, it has a vanishingly low profile. There is mild bemusement at sporadic excursions of medical students who wander the locale searching for the landmarks of *A Fortunate Man*. A few grumbles can be heard among the old families about the book's depiction of the population here as 'culturally deprived' foresters: 'The village was a bit unhappy about it, because I think Berger exaggerated that underclass part of it.' There are also a handful of residents proud to point out their relatives among the book's photographs: 'My sister and her boyfriend are in one of the pictures at the dance' or 'That's my grandfather there, the grey-haired chap.' There is one ninety-nine-year-old lady, now housebound, who appears as a lithe young woman, photographed by Jean Mohr on Sassall's consulting couch, her skirt pulled high above her pale knees. 'There was a lot of hoo-ha about that,' says her son-in-law. 'My wife's grandmother, oh she went bananas, being in a book like that, but I think she's quite chuffed to think that she's in it now.'

All the same, the abiding memories tend to relate not to the 1967 book, but to the doctor himself, who cared for his patients here from the late 1940s until the early 1980s. These recollections tend to revolve around a few key themes: Dr John's early flair for dramatic medical rescues, followed by his later all-consuming dedication to his patients, as well as a lifelong habit of swearing like a sailor and occasional episodes of flamboyant eccentricity. After the initial tales of roadside amputations and kitchen table appendicectomies, there came more than one account of a sickly infant relieved of a dangerous fever on Christmas Day, midnight summons to the surgery to avert anaphylaxis, babies delivered (he apparently hated to leave any birth to the midwife), elders tenderly waited upon in their final hours, and villagers pulled up by the doctor in the lane because he'd noticed they didn't look well. One neighbour and close friend can remember telling her son, 'For God's sake, don't tell John you've got a headache, or he'll be round here,' and sure enough he was, whipping the child away to have electrodes placed on his temples.

In tandem with this crushing sense of responsibility for the health of the entire community ran a bruising candour. Several spoke of Dr John's 'plain-speaking', his impatience with malingerers and forthright love of a cuss-word. 'His language got a bit strong sometimes, mind,' said one old man, who clearly thought there no finer doctor anywhere in the world, 'but that's how he was, you know, he told you straight.'

The other vein of affectionate reminiscence that has endured the forty years since Dr John's demise relates to instances of his extravagant theatricality and his energy. Take the occasion Dr John undertook his home visits in full equestrian apparel, bareback on a neighbour's pony, which duly nibbled and trampled each patient's lettuces and sweet peas in turn. Or there was his decision to rid the village of a plague of jackdaws, whereupon the family gardener was recruited to drive Dr John around, this time costumed with safari suit and shotgun, as he fired at the pestilent corvids through the open window of his Land Rover, a neighbour's children scampering behind with a sack for the dead birds. The zeal with which he mobilized every man and boy to help clear, drain and replant the derelict moat of the small castle in the centre of the village is immortalized in a sun-drenched cinefilm. Filmed by Dr John himself, it is full of men in flat caps, sickles and rakes in hand. From time to time, his wife, Betty, takes over the camera and he pads into shot in a woollen navvy's hat, a fag on and Hector the family hound at his heel, as he heaves a rock here, straightens the angle of a pump there. He exudes purpose, and something that looks like happiness. Late in his career, Dr John spent a few months in China, learning the rudiments of acupuncture from the barefoot doctors of the rural hinterlands, and on his return was to be seen about the village in Mao-style tunic suit and cap, keen to practise his new art on anyone who would let him. A close family friend told me that she sometimes looks back and wonders whether these flourishes of chameleon exuberance, not to mention the ripe language, operated like a safety valve for the intense responsibility he felt for every man, woman and child on his patient list, many of whom he knew like the back of his hand.

His son put it like this: 'My father was a man of many masks, and not only in dress. There was his Medical mask for dealing with patients and medical colleagues, his Village Squire mask, which enabled him to mix freely with the gentry, but also farmers and labourers, his Urbane Intellectual mask, because he was very well read and could talk Freud or Conrad with the likes of Berger. Finally there was his Family mask, primarily for dealing with us three kids. We could never get behind this mask, which was probably just as well, because I think the man behind it would have scared us. Betty, our mother, was the only person to get behind all the masks, or to see which mask was in place and to support and protect him whatever. She was the only one who could recognize when he was suicidal and could, on three occasions that I was aware of, then pre-empt the actual act. But she wasn't around for the fourth.'

A Fortunate Man refers to the episodes of depression that periodically assail Sassall and manifest through a fixation on the welfare of his patients coupled with a sense of his own inadequacy in the face of their suffering. What emerges from speaking with those who knew the real Dr John is that this depression had always been part of his life, and that in the years after the book was written, it worsened. Indeed, it's no secret that he's believed to have suffered from what is now termed bipolar disorder, referred to in the past as 'manic depression'. He endured ECT treatment in hospital, which he loathed and swore made no difference. He also attempted suicide on a number of occasions, each averted by his wife, Betty, who became skilled at spotting the signs of a dangerous decline.

Which is why one notable omission in Berger's *A Fortunate Man* is so problematic, and some would say unforgivable. For the doctor's wife, Betty, was simply written out of it. She makes just a brief appearance in the dedication and in a single footnote: 'I do not attempt in this essay to discuss the role of Sassall's wife or his children. My concern is his professional life.' This infuriated friends and family who knew that, given the nature of the community and the doctor's role within it, the distinction was specious. Practising medicine in a place like this, at a time like that, the boundaries between professional and personal were highly porous. Moreover, Betty played a pivotal role, not just emotionally and domestically, but also professionally. She ran the surgery, kept the books and dispensed medications, as well as endeavouring to keep the doctor in one piece. It was commonplace for a patient to say to Betty, 'Oh those tablets Dr John gave me made me bad' or 'The pain has come back, Betty', and she would mediate between doctor and patient, an intrinsic part of the very relationship the book set out to explore. Berger had painted Sassall as a lone Conradian figure, a 'master mariner', but in reality the good ship Sassall was kept afloat as much by Betty as by its troubled captain.

Betty's closest confidante through those years still lives in the same long, low stone cottage, heavy with roses and honeysuckle. It lies on the steep lane behind John and Betty's old house, with its fine chimneys and mullioned windows that gaze out across a broad reach of the valley. For fifteen years, the two families were the firmest of friends. John had delivered her daughter in the bedroom upstairs, causing much hilarity by serving the afterbirth in a casserole dish from her own kitchen to the family dog. 'He was a wonderful character,' she said. 'Erratic, eccentric, exciting, and also the most brilliant doctor, the way he related to people, he was really caring. But he did have these incredible mood swings and when the black dog came, it would totally tip him over. John was a very, very clever man, and Betty was even cleverer. I always used to say that he was a Greek and she was a Roman, in that she was practical and he wasn't; he was a muser. Betty was his guardian angel, really. She would ring me up and say, "John's depressed, please can you have the gun?", and I would go over to fetch it and lock it up here under the stairs. I mean, he had access to drugs all the time, but Betty, she'd be watching him like a hawk. Pretty well everyone round here was aware that he struggled from time to time, but although he was depressed, he was still the *patrón*, if you understand what I mean. He was like the head man or the priest. People were immensely fond of them both, you see? They were both *patrónes*, John and Betty.'

In 1981, aged sixty-one, Betty suffered a sudden, catastrophic heart attack and died. Without her, Dr John unravelled. 'I think he realized he was spinning out of control without Betty,' their old friend said. 'He was becoming more eccentric and his young partners at the practice were encouraging him to retire. I think he thought, *What shall I do now? It's been my life, it is my life, my practice is me.* He was alone, he was adrift. Then he retired and we had a retirement party in the moat. There was a huge crowd of people there, his oldest patient and his youngest, lots to eat and drink. I think probably that was when he thought, *That's it now. I'm no longer the doctor.* And that made his life very empty, no Betty, no practice. I'd said to my husband, when Betty died, "I don't think John will last long" and that's exactly what happened.'

THE WINTER AFTER Betty's death was the coldest on record in this part of the country. Worse even than the year they'd arrived, the valley was muffled by snowdrifts for many weeks on end. Dr John retired just as spring fought through and the periwinkles and primroses at the edge of the woods began to bloom. His leaving party was in April, but not even the redemptive abundance of the summer that followed, fattening the valley below his house into a soft billow of green, could avert what many deemed inevitable. His friends and family could not watch him for every hour of every day, and by mid-August, it was too late.

Dr John's obituary in the *British Medical Journal* in the autumn of 1982 does not mention that he took his own life. It simply signs off with the line, 'An indefatigable worker, he was dogged by ill health over the past 15 years, and his wife's death in 1981 hastened his own.' Some years later, John Berger added an afterword to *A Fortunate Man*. 'I do not search for what I might have foreseen and didn't,' he wrote, 'as if the essential was missing from what passed between us; rather I now begin with his violent death, and, from it, look back with increased tenderness on what he set out to do and what he offered to others, for as long as he could endure.'

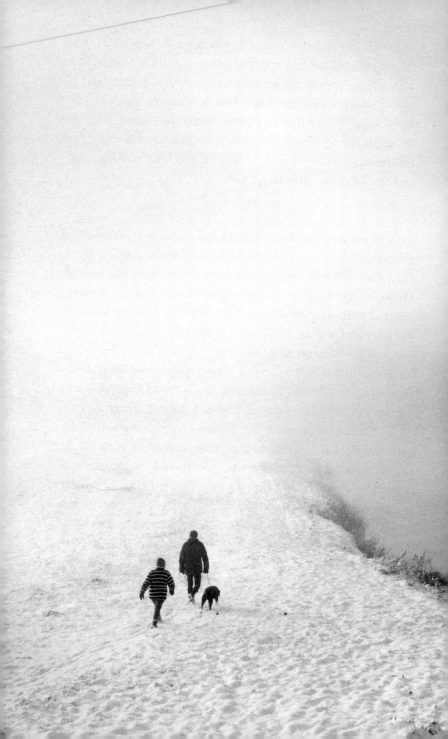

Now SILVER-HAIRED and in retirement, one of the young doctors who worked with Dr John from the early 1970s, and through the last nine turbulent years of his life, considers his legacy from the most intimate of standpoints. 'I was thinking about John this morning and in today's medicine, he wouldn't have lasted. He'd have been drummed out because of his eccentricity, but what he taught me was a totally different way of looking at general practice and medicine and people. He was one of very few GPs at that time who were light years ahead.'

It is a distinctive feature of small rural practices, such as this one, that there can emerge a familial pattern of inheritance from one generation of doctors to the next. With each successive generation, there are naturally disagreements, departures from the old ways, new directions taken, just as in any family, but there is also a built-in mechanism for the passage of ideas from hand to hand. Or so it has been here in the valley.

'I'd come with a fairly narrow, restrictive medical training, very structured and hierarchical, and all of a sudden I arrived with John and I'm thinking, *Blimey, can you do that?* It left me floundering to begin with, but what he taught me was that caring for people and the art of medicine was about much more than just sitting there and giving people pills, or cutting them open and sewing them back up again. It truly was an art. It required a much more expansive idea of being a human being, rather than just being somebody with a medical degree on the wall who's dishing out pills. I'd already done some of that seeing-forty-five-people-in-a-morning-surgery and found that you can't really achieve very much, but when I came to this practice, there was time to sit and talk to people. This is one of the essential things about rural practice, the fact that you're part of a community. It was John who taught me that and that caring for people was about listening to them, understanding them, trying to put yourself in their shoes, accepting each person for who they are, recognizing them as a person. Because that's important to people and it's part of the broader context of good health. So that's what John gave me, and it's one of the things that's so essential about general practice that's now in danger of being lost.'

After Dr John's death, this young doctor would go on to serve another quarter of a century in the green folds of the valley. For the last six of his thirty-four years here, he was joined by a young female GP. She was never his trainee – he takes pains to point out that she arrived a fully qualified colleague – but he did, he admits, 'dispense a few pearls of wisdom, such as they are'. In turn, she came to look upon him as a mentor, who taught her much about the practice of medicine in a place like this. Just as you can grow to resemble a grandparent you have never met, so she in time would grow to embody some of the ideals of Dr John. She had moved a few years earlier with her fiancé into a small cottage in a hamlet directly across the valley from Dr John's former home. From over his garden wall, you could just make out the whitewashed stone of her home, framed by woodland and a paddock below, the fortunate man's last view a new beginning for the fortunate woman.

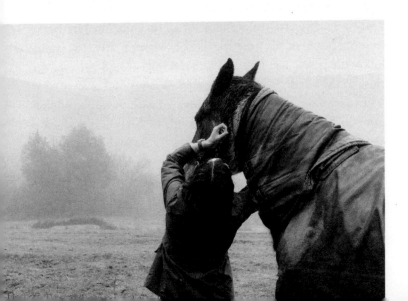

EXACTLY A DECADE EARLIER, she had started at medical school in London. The pastoral solitude and intensive revision of her sixth-form years meant that she arrived in the big city, aged eighteen, like a coiled spring. Determined to cram all the adventure and romance she'd expected of adolescence into those last two years of her teens, she had set about London life at full tilt. There were parties, and lots of them, friendships, love. There were January days spent not in the lecture hall, where she should have been, but freezing in a cardboard box outside the US Embassy, protesting the first Gulf War. She hurled herself at everything this glorious new freedom had to offer, with the possible exception of a scrupulous attendance to her studies. Imagining the intelligence that had fetched up a pristine set of A levels would carry her through again, she soon found out that she was wrong. She failed several end-of-year papers. There followed an excruciating summer preparing for retakes in September. She can still remember her terror the night before results day, her lament to friends that she'd be thrown out, that her life and all her dreams were over. One of them had laughed and said she was being 'emotionally extravagant', that she'd be fine, which of course she was, and the second of five years' training to become a junior doctor began – but it was a wake-up call. She really did want to be a doctor. Her heart had told her first, but now she thought about it, hard, her head followed. It was the first and last time she would ever sail so close to the wind.

In the summer of 1995, she graduated with the top medicine prize in her year. Now the real work of becoming a doctor began, not in theory, but in practice. By now she was highly ambitious, which made her suggestible to the dominant narrative of aspiration towards a hospital specialism. Yes, she'd loved her work experience in general practice as a sixth-former, and her GP attachment as a student, but she couldn't help thinking she was a little too good for this cosy, cardiganed branch of medicine. There was glamour and dynamism in hospital work, more intellectual challenge, she was sure, more life-and-death drama, more heroics. So she set aside any idea of following the example of Dr Sassall in the book that had so bewitched her at the age of seventeen, and she dived headlong into two years of placements as a hospital junior doctor. Maybe she'd be a psychiatrist, maybe a paediatrician, perhaps even a surgeon. The world was waiting for her.

THE SENIOR REGISTRAR in the surgery department had been shouting at her for the better part of ten weeks. The senior reg was a formidable woman, who had fought her way into one of the more macho of hospital specialisms, and appeared to believe that a jolly good beasting was essential to the induction of a young doctor. She seemed to have taken a particular dislike to the mousy-haired, wide-eyed and studiously conscientious junior doctor currently working on her team. Perhaps she was irritated by the way the young woman absorbed her opprobrium day after day, like blotting paper, simply trying harder, making ever longer lists on her clipboard of what she had to do and stoically working through them, ticking each one off, double-checking and triple-checking, in a futile attempt to avoid the next torrent of disdain. For that was how the newly minted doctor had learned to mediate difficulty: with hard, hard work. All the same, she'd not had a noisy childhood and couldn't bear shouting. It wasn't that she lacked backbone, but she always found herself disconcerted by outright aggression. It was not how she did business.

These attritional volleys of hostility never took place behind closed doors. Instead they were unleashed at high volume in the middle of the ward, surrounded by patients in their beds, as if humiliation were a valuable teaching tool and a soothing entertainment for the mortally ill. That morning, the shouting pertained to a scan that the senior registrar said was needed for the very poorly elderly lady in Bed 7, whom the young doctor had been looking after for several days. She had already been down to radiology to request it, but had been refused by the consultant, whereupon she'd returned and been barked at. Back she had fled, down the three flights of stairs to radiology, with a better story and a certain desperation in her demeanour, but again she'd been rebuffed. Upon receiving this news, delivered at a terrified murmur, the senior registrar had flown into a rage at the patient's bedside. At the top of her lungs, she castigated the young doctor for her stupidity, her ineptitude, her pathetic time-wasting. What was wrong with her? How would she ever succeed as a doctor if she couldn't complete a task that any fool could accomplish with their eyes closed? On and on it went. The young doctor did not move, her shame overflowing. Tears welled and began to fall, one by one, onto the blue linoleum at her feet. The old lady in Bed 7 didn't say a word, but through the salty blur, the young house officer saw her arm stir and reach up towards her. She felt the small, bony hand at the very end of its days slip into her own and squeeze it firmly. For almost a minute, they held hands, doctor and patient, until the shouting had run its course. The old lady in Bed 7 died two days later.

Had this scalding experience not been preceded by six happy months working in general medicine and geriatrics, the doctor says she would have quit medicine there and then. As it was, she progressed to the next house officer post in orthopaedics, where she felt valued again, able to do what was expected of her, and managed to rehabilitate her love for the job. Still, the new doctor's mortification at the episode, her sense that they had let a dying woman down, stayed with her, and it taught her a number of vital lessons about the kind of doctor she wanted to be. One: if a patient is comforting you, when you should be comforting them, then there is something seriously wrong with how you are working. Two: workplace bullying, overt or subtle, is always damaging to both doctor and patient. Three: the relationship with patients, its mutuality, matters, and it mattered to her more than almost anything else; in the future she must always try to fight for it. Four: people, even at the very brink of life, are amazing. You forget that at your peril.

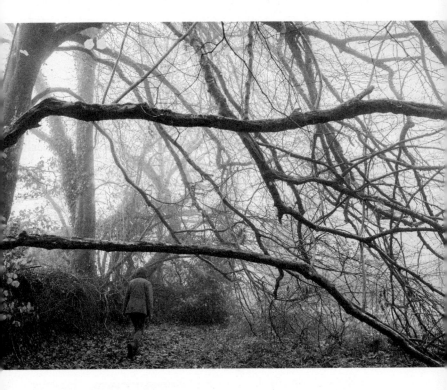

THE TWO WOMEN are in their mid-twenties, the mother of the child and the young doctor now over halfway through her clinical training, although the limpid quality of youth is on the wane for them both. For one woman, three years of motherhood is to blame, for the other, three years as a junior doctor. They have in common punishing hours, chronic sleep deprivation and a weight of responsibility that's obliged them to grow up fast, although this is no time to discuss any of that. The child, squirming and whining on his mother's lap, is their sole concern. They share that too.

It's an ear infection, she tells the mother, having taken a full history and conducted a thorough examination of the fretful, feverish toddler. Earache can be very unpleasant for little ones, she explains, as the child is tucked back into his clothes and clipped into the pushchair, ready for the journey home across the city. The young doctor is just organizing the antibiotics from the hospital pharmacy, when the mother speaks.

'Was this rash here before?'

The woman has crooked her finger into the neckline of her son's T-shirt to reveal a patch of red pinprick spots spreading like a stain on the child's neck and shoulder. The doctor's stomach lurches.

No, she says, let's have another look.

As they ease the now screaming child back out of his T-shirt and trousers on the bed, the doctor can see a classic meningococcal rash appearing with alarming speed: first chest and back, now arms, legs and face, the spots expanding into reddish blotches before their eyes.

'Jesus,' says the mother, 'what *is* that?'

From across the hospital campus, the two women can hear the wail of a siren stop as an ambulance swings into the emergency bay. The doctor can sense the mother's breathing

74

quicken. Hers has too, though she hopes to God the other woman cannot tell. She feels out of her depth.

Alright, she says, I see. Her tone is a deliberate calm that she's not at all sure is convincing. I think we should see what the consultant thinks. He's doing the ward round now. Just sit tight for a moment.

With all the haste she can muster without breaking into a run, she walks to the nurses' station, murmurs a few words and a nurse rushes to find the consultant. She returns to the mother and child, but relinquishes the emergency almost immediately, when the consultant strides into the room and takes control. She retreats to the staff toilet at the end of the corridor, locks the door, and weeps convulsively at how close she came to getting this wrong. Then she splashes cold water on her face, mopping it with a rough paper towel until she looks more or less presentable, takes a deep, deep breath and returns to the next poorly child and worried parent.

The little boy with meningitis spends the next ten days in the paediatric intensive-care unit. There are junctures when it's not certain he'll survive and the young doctor finds herself more than once crying in a lavatory cubicle at the sheer terror of the work she has chosen. But in years to come, she will look back on days like these as a gruelling but essential apprenticeship in managing fear, indeed in managing all her emotions.

THERE IS A LOT of fear in a doctor's work. Call it stress or pressure if you prefer, but in the early days of learning one's trade as a medic, it is often just good old-fashioned terror: plain, simple, white-knuckled. The young doctor had acquired a certain blueprint for handling fear early in life, one that she says she 'learnt from the best'. Where her father instilled optimism, it was her mother who always evinced an almost superhuman capacity for calm. Throughout the doctor's childhood, her young mother managed to retain both her composure and an ability to make measured, effective decisions through an assortment of rural emergencies. There was the great storm that threatened to rip the roof off the family farm, saved only by judicious use of ropes and breeze blocks to lash the building to the hill, as one might secure cargo on the deck of a ship. There were the almost annual birthing emergencies with cows and horses, their young snagged halfway into the world. There was even a broken horsebox on the M4 in the middle of a thunderstorm, where in order to fix the vehicle, three racehorses had to be unloaded onto the hard shoulder as the lightning flashed. It's perhaps not surprising that the doctor's mother retrained as a nurse once her daughter had left for medical school. She eventually qualified as an advanced neonatal nurse practitioner, and to this day cares for dangerously ill babies during transit by air ambulance. She's temperamentally suited to this work; nothing ruffles her.

As for her daughter, she had grown up observing this capacity for grace under pressure. She knew what it looked like, even if it didn't come naturally to her at first. In time, the heightened passions of her university years, that 'emotional extravagance' about which her friends had teased her, gave way to something more nuanced. The intensity of feeling was still there, as compelling as ever, but she was learning to lever an air gap between emotion and the action necessary in a crisis. This was a chance discovery at first, some spontaneous, intuitive simulation of her mother's studied calm, but finding that it worked and helped her do the job, it was a behaviour that the doctor then cultivated in herself. Nearly twenty-five years later, it is one of the aspects of her personality that her colleagues in the valley practice mention again and again: how very calm she is, no matter what is going on.

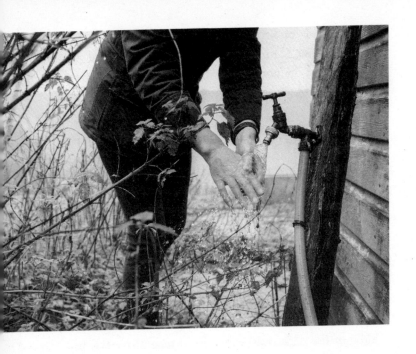

THE HOSPITAL BUILDING had the quality of a manifesto about it. The heroic modernism of its concrete bulk, conceived when the NHS was in its infancy, suggested a future in which the vagaries of human suffering would be overmastered by the great machine of modern science. A vast facade of 637 identical windows, arranged in seven long rows, cast their medical gaze towards the city, whose sick it promised to deliver by the thousand. The building was designed in the late 1950s by a serial contestant in architectural competitions, his radical blueprints for Coventry Cathedral and the Sydney Opera House having been turned down. Construction wasn't completed until over a decade later, several years after the architect's death. The Queen opened the hospital in the winter of 1971, three weeks before the junior doctor, intermittently given to weeping in the staff toilets there, was born.

These kinds of brutalist monoliths were already growing passé when Her Majesty's white-gloved hand pulled the little rope to unveil the commemorative plaque. By the late 1990s, the bleak slab of the main hospital building was surrounded by a sprawling campus of smaller modern blocks and car parks. Attempts had been made to enliven the area with a few shrubs, saplings and a desultory rectangle or two of scraggy grass, but mostly it was about long, narrow pavements and high walls, adorned only with humming air-conditioning units, access gantries and an occasional fire door. The young doctor hated it. That 1959 architectural vision of modernity and equality came across to her, forty-odd years later, as a dystopian uniformity. It seemed out of step with the respect for the individual that she'd been taught was central in modern medicine. That, and the fact that sprinting half a mile across the deserted campus from the junior doctors' block when the on-call crash bleep went in the middle of the night was scary. She'd taken to carrying a rape alarm and her uncle had given her a canister of some dubious spray, just in case.

She had been desperate to get this job. It was oversubscribed and the interview was tough, so she was overjoyed when they offered her the sought-after position on the children's ward. Paediatrics was, at this point, what she thought she wanted to do. She'd always loved working with children, and recognized from previous paediatric placements that this specialism entailed more continuity of care than many. Sick children and their families would return time and again, both in outpatients and on the wards, and the young doctor relished these longer relationships pieced together over numerous encounters.

Thus she began with the highest of hopes and was to spend two years working here. The hours were hard, fifty-six-hour shifts, during which she'd sleep, patchily, on site. She learned to cope with that, more or less, but what proved harder to stomach was the conveyor-belt culture of this particular department, very different from anywhere she'd worked before. Here no one seemed to know your name, or had time for much in the way of individual teaching. Of course, she learned a huge amount, and says today she wouldn't have missed the experience for the world – this woman is wired to find the silver lining in any cloud – but that sense of being a tiny, anonymous cog in a vast machine did not suit her temperament. Not at all.

She had grown up a good deal since those epiphanies of her late teenage years – the leveret! the song! the book! – but that didn't mean she couldn't still be swayed by a powerfully instinctive form of resolve. It was not that she saw the world in black and white. She didn't. She knew that much of life is lived in the grey areas, but something about her vivid emotional engagement with the present, the very character trait that made her an empathic doctor, also predisposed her to a kind of acute-onset decision-making.

The subliminal misgivings about the job burst into the foreground at the end of a long, long shift, towards the end of her second year. She'd been on call all night, back and forth across the mugger's paradise of the concrete campus, caring for a young girl with type 1 diabetes whose blood sugar kept plummeting dangerously. That night, she hadn't been to bed at all. The following lunchtime she was called into the consultant's office and told she would also have to cover the next night, as a colleague had phoned in sick. There had been much staff absence recently, perhaps because of the caustic culture of the department, and management had decided that any further sick days would be covered not by locums but by the team themselves. It was collective punishment of a sort. The young doctor explained to the consultant that she couldn't cover that night. Her cat was unwell and she had a vet's appointment, but the consultant was having none of it. He stood in front of the door, barring her way out. 'But I covered last night,' she said, visibly upset, 'I'm exhausted.' That was not his problem, he said, these were the rules and she was not leaving the office until she'd agreed to do it. She duly worked the second night, but something had snapped. The following morning she turned to the vacancies page of the *British Medical Journal*, saw a GP training job not far away and applied there and then. The interview was the next afternoon. By the third day, she'd resigned, and before long left the many-eyed behemoth of a building for the last time.

Anyone who's ever worked in A&E, or in any other branch of medicine for that matter, knows that life can, and regularly does, turn on a sixpence. It would perhaps make for a neater story if this young doctor's transition from paediatrics to primary care had not been one of those on-a-sixpence moments, and had instead been driven by cool-headed, vocational strategy. Yet within what might seem an arbitrary, impetuous decision – exhaustion, an ailing cat, a mean boss, an unlovely building – lies the very essence of why she would turn out to be so well suited to her new life, indeed why she has more in common with the doctor in *A Fortunate Man* than is at first apparent.

That willingness to invest in the moment, that instinctive ability to occupy, reflect and respond to the here and now, both emotionally and intellectually, sits at the heart of the doctor–patient relationship as it plays out in general practice. Where the scalpel is the essential instrument of the surgeon, so the relationship is the instrument of the general practitioner. Building good relationships calls for both spontaneity and judgement. Summoning afresh, in each ten-minute increment, empathy, precision, collaborative decision-making and shrewd risk management, requires an ability to wipe the blackboard clean with each encounter. It is about looking and listening with the utmost care, wringing every verbal and non-verbal vestige of meaning from those scarce 600 seconds; then, if you are lucky enough to have a high proportion of long-standing patients, to knit it all together over time. It is a job that requires both heart and head. The young doctor, now a trainee GP, finally found herself able to use both as never before, no longer in opposition with one another, but in delicate balance. Even today, more than two decades on, to watch her with patients is to observe gusts of emotion and fellow feeling, humour or concern, blow across her face, like weather moving across a landscape.

Spring begins in the valley from the ground up.

While the sky is still leaden and the branches bare, the air damp and cold, while mist still clings to the river and the banter of mufflered kids at the school bus stop forms airborne boughs of breath above their heads, rebirth commences discreetly at the forest floor. To the casual glance at either landscape or calendar, it's winter still, but across the steep woods, colour stirs. The moss and lichen that carpets every rock, every wall, wraps itself about the ankles of every tree, begins to glow, a vibrant, graphic, emerald green. Long before the daffodils and bluebells that appear on postcards make their entrance, this uncanny viridescence is a calling card of the coming season, a totem of renewal, legible only to those who live here.

For centuries now, the valley has had two faces that gaze in opposite directions, like Janus himself. One face is turned outward to the world, drawing in visitors during the warmer months. Eager to partake of nature's majesty, they are easy to spot, searching for the picture-postcard bluebell woods on their OS maps, posting the view on Instagram or picnicking in Arcadian fashion on the riverbank, to the fury of local fishermen. Two hundred years ago or more, there were poets, painters and assorted aesthetes who did much the same. They flocked here in search of the sublime, and were most handsomely rewarded by the crags and the mists and the woods, by the bosky peasants and their exquisite, half-ruined dwellings. Now there are Lycra-clad pelotons of urban cyclists instead, who annoy the residents all summer long, their fitness objectives clogging the traffic on the road that winds with the river from one end of the gorge to the other. The financial realities of small-scale agriculture and cottage industry are such that it's harder to earn your crust these days by sending the fruits of your labours and land out into the world; it's more viable to bring people in. So there are paddleboarders and wild swimmers too, drone pilots, canoeists and glum troupes of backpacked teenagers earning their Duke of Edinburgh's Awards. Each of these elicits a roll of the eye from the people who live here and prefer to keep their valley to themselves. 'It's like a recreation area,' complains one. 'A big park, you know? Day trippers, Airbnb an' all that.'

But the valley has another face, a private one that it saves for its own. These are its lovelier and more subtle joys, the fleeting ones that sightseers miss, for they reward the accustomed senses. The bright February moss is one such, but there are many: the trio of young stags that struts past the kitchen window chewing stolen apples; the glow-worm that pulses nocturnal signals from the crevices of the garden wall still hot from the day's sun; the nightjars that churr and click in the cryptic dusk of still, warm evenings on the heathland above the river; the oceanic roar of the woods in a storm; the hidden paths so rarely traversed that, by winter, ornate traceries of spiderwebs freeze across them, like baroque gates; the spectral skein of mist they call 'The White Lady' that drifts and coils above the waters of the river; the great sea of an autumn fog from which the uplands of the valley protrude, an archipelago sketched in pencil. These are the gifts that capture and hold the hearts of the people for whom this place is home. They mark time and change and continuity. This is the relationship between landscape and people at its most intimate.

THE ACT OF PARLIAMENT that paved the way for the designation and protection of this valley as an Area of Outstanding Natural Beauty was part of the same legislative programme of post-war reconstruction that created the National Health Service. Passed the following year, the 1949 National Parks and Access to the Countryside Act was seen as complementary to the new NHS, a means to promote good mental and physical health through exercise and the enjoyment of nature. To live in one, while serving the other, had a pleasing symmetry that was not lost on the now fully qualified doctor, as she weighed up her first professional move as a general practitioner.

She had first visited this valley while still a junior doctor in London, having fallen in love with a young man who'd grown up nearby. She remembers stopping with him at the village stores on the green valley road on that very first visit. A small boy had come in to ask the shopkeeper for advice as to what to feed a rook he'd found with a broken wing. The man had taken the enquiry very seriously, fetching some injured rook food from the storeroom and devoting some minutes to a discussion of the optimal conditions for rook convalescence. There was no charge for the food and no one in the queue batted an eyelid at waiting to pay while the matter was dealt with. The young doctor duly fell head over heels in love with the valley too, the twin romances entwining. She could breathe here; she could think; she felt both free and protected the moment the road left the town at one end of the valley, and turned steeply into the tangled woods. A few years later, in the spring, the young couple bought their first home together, a whitewashed stone cottage with a little paddock for a horse, set into the hillside above the river. The following summer, with flowers in her hair, she and her father rode by pony and trap down the steep hill from the cottage to the village church. There she was married, not three minutes' walk from the doctor's surgery where she would soon decide to spend the rest of her working life – although she didn't know it yet.

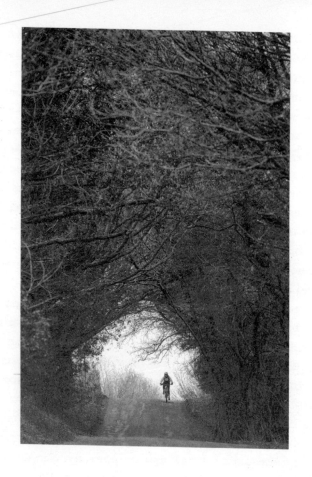

THE ADVERTISEMENT WAS for a part-time salaried doctor, just three surgeries a week, in the local practice with its twin outposts either side of the river. So she applied for it, in tandem with another three-quarter-time GP role in a town practice fifteen miles away. In the three years they'd been living in the valley, she'd undertaken a handful of hospital jobs around the county in order to sign off her training, but here was an opportunity to mesh work and life together. Many general practitioners actively prefer not to do this, favouring a substantial commute over the goldfish bowl insularity of caring for the community in which they live. The concern is chiefly about 'boundaries'. How can a doctor be both a friend and neighbour at the same time as being one's physician? And if that plural role is possible, is it healthy? There are other caveats attached to working in a small, rural practice – the difficulty of finding locum cover, the potential isolation and, back then in 2000, the likelihood of greater on-call commitments at all hours of the day and night – but the lack of anonymity is the thing that makes a good many doctors shudder. The prospect of being unable to walk the dog without someone ambushing you with their latest symptom, or the impossibility of nipping to the shop without the oven chips and wine in your trolley drawing comment, would be hell for some. Yet for this doctor, it seemed a price worth paying for that sense of rootedness which had always eluded her. Here was a chance to bed down within a close community, both making a difference there and making it home. Besides, she knew by now that she craved continuity professionally too, that the better she knew her patients the more this grounded her clinical practice in something that felt warm and human, and that this, in turn, enhances the care a doctor is able to give.

And so, as the air took on a tinge of autumn chill, the rich green of the summer woods now flecked with yellow and the sound of the wind through the leaves more sibilant, the doctor began at the valley practice.

She was to be working alongside the one-time partner of Dr John, the 'fortunate man' himself; not that she realized it. It was the future of the practice she and the older doctor discussed over sandwich lunches, not the past, and she'd half forgotten about Berger's book anyway, having no idea at the time that it concerned her own little corner of Eden. For these were turbulent years for their profession. Some months earlier, a provincial GP, Dr Harold Shipman, had been convicted of the murder of fifteen of his female patients and was believed to have been responsible for the deaths of up to 250 more. The trial and ensuing public inquiry led to a host of changes in medical procedure, practice and oversight. It was another nail in the coffin for the old-school paternalism of which Dr Sassall had been the benign apotheosis, and Shipman the abominable nadir. Models of trust within the doctor–patient relationship shifted towards a more equal footing between doctor and patient, now expected to work in collaboration, side by side rather than simply face to face. Although not directly related to what became known as 'the Shipman Effect', a revised GP contract was negotiated in 2004, and that marked the end of doctors' 24-hour responsibility for their patients. The task of organizing weekend and night-time care now moved to an out-of-hours service and a new era for the family doctor began, one that would be unrecognizable (and one suspects unconscionable) to Dr John. Yet she, his medical heir apparent, understood that the seasons change, the world turns, and that if she was to be part of this next generation of general practitioners, it was no good mourning an age now dead and gone. Instead, she would have to remake the country doctor in her own image, preserving as much as she could of what was valuable from the old world, but also keeping pace with the new.

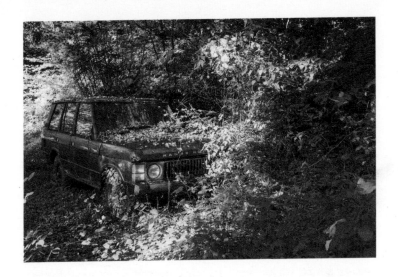

THESE EARLY YEARS in the valley were all about finding her way as a doctor – in every sense of the word. Indeed, in the days before satnav and decent mobile phone coverage, she spent a good deal of her home-visit time getting lost.

There are no streets as such in this part of the world, just a labyrinth of unmarked green lanes with hedges that bulge in summer, narrow stone walls, and grasses that grow high in the middle of the road. There's little logic to their convolutions, bifurcations and occasional surprising dead ends, where the lane simply forgets itself and peters out, leaving your headlights glaring into the trees. Addresses are generally nothing more than the name of the house, the name of the village and a postcode, although don't for a minute suppose that this helps much, even in the age of Google Maps. Many of the postcodes cut perverse slices down the steep valley sides, with houses ten minutes' drive apart sharing the same unhelpful seven characters, while the village boundaries enjoy a whimsy all their own. Indeed, several of the smaller hamlets have no identifying signage whatsoever. To compound the matter, the houses themselves often have no name on the gate, so it's entirely routine to arrive at your destination with little idea as to whether you're in the right place at all. The locals have always secretly loved it, this arcane geography that confounds outsiders, but for the fresh-faced young doctor newly arrived at the surgery, they willingly made an exception. She learned to ask patients if they might leave an upstairs light on, or sling a towel over the gate, perhaps activate the hazard lights on their car, so that she could find them.

This navigational ordeal for the new doctor was only heightened by the archaic dimensions of the byways, more suited to carts and horses than motor vehicles. Frequently, the execution of a forty-three-point turn in a narrow track would see an overgrown stone trough, a tree stump or an uneven wall knock a dent in her bumper. It's an item of faith in the valley that one ceases to care too much about dents. Still, a few alarming experiences with patients (typically elderly and male) who at the end of the visit would hobble out to 'see her back', taught the young doctor to turn the car around on arrival, in order to facilitate an easy exit.

That wasn't possible the night she was called to a patient she'd never met before. The man had recently been diagnosed with lung cancer and had moved back from the city to his holiday house while he came to terms with a bleak prognosis. His notes were still in transit from his registered doctor, so when she arrived at the house that night, in driving rain and after several wrong turns in the woods, the doctor knew only the barest outline of his situation. The gravel in front of the house was already jammed with cars – his extended family had gathered in the teeth of the emergency – so she had pulled in at an angle, left the keys on the dashboard, and hurried inside. There followed a gruelling consultation. The man was breathless and scared, in a fierce state of denial as to the severity of his condition, and with only a couple of pieces of paperwork to account for what was going on. She had nothing from the oncologist, nothing from his previous doctor. She had to piece it together, with the man pausing to cough up blood, his wife tugging in panic at her sleeve with conflicting fragments of information, and the melee of concerned relatives murmuring in the hall outside. She was with the man for a long time. As she finally emerged into the wet night, emotionally spent, a young man called to her from the light of the open door.

'Thank you, doctor, thank you so much.' His voice quivered. She noticed he looked like a younger version of the dying man indoors. 'I hope you don't mind. I turned your car around, so you could get out.'

She thanked him.

'And I gave it a quick wash too. I hope you don't think that's rude. I just wanted to do something, and—'

She smiled. 'Go on, say it.'

'And I've never seen such a dirty white car.'

For a moment, the two of them laughed together, as the rain fell.

The joys of this work, she was beginning to realize, did not only come from the lighter moments. She was growing to love this job.

WHEN SHE HAD BEEN a year or so in the role, the doctor's husband, still in his twenties, suffered a protracted spell of serious illness. Suddenly at the sharp end of medical care, she attended his numerous hospital appointments whenever she could. It was a terrifying time, and to stave off the worry of those waiting-room hours, she found herself reading more than she had in years. Books had always been a refuge for her, but finding it hard to concentrate, she now turned to her comfort reading of old, *Black Beauty*, *I Capture the Castle*, *The Bone People*. Searching her shelves one day for another reassuring favourite, she spotted the second-hand copy of *A Fortunate Man* she'd bought as a sixth-former. She had reread it twice since then, once at medical school during her GP rotation and again during her registrar training. Each time, the story of Dr Sassall had taught her something new about the central mystery of medical practice: the relationship between illness and the whole person, the affliction and the afflicted. She had come to know, first-hand, that understanding and honouring that relationship lay at the heart of a doctor's work. She also now understood what she hadn't as a teenager: that the story was not just about one obscure country physician, but touched something universal in the experience of doctors and their patients everywhere. It was a book that, however melancholy, always felt redemptive to her, if only because the central character himself was such a fundamentally good man and a good doctor. It was the perfect read for a time like this. She took *A Fortunate Man* down from the shelf and slipped it into her bag to read at the hospital later that day, certain it would make her feel better.

The realization, sitting there on the stiff plastic chair in the waiting room, was almost physical. She'd been thumbing through the book, distracted, looking at the photographs, when, with a jolt, she spotted the final image in the book.

The photograph shows the 1960s doctor, in tweed jacket and cords, his back to the camera, trudging his incongruously polished black shoes up a steep, overgrown path to a white cottage. The boughs of a small orchard, heavy with fruit, frame him. At the top of the grassy path, in a dark dress and long white apron, the tiny figure of a woman watches the doctor's approach, her hand raised to wave hello or to shield her eyes from the bright sky reflected in the cottage windows behind her.

She flinched. She knew that cottage, that path. She knew those apple trees. On a home visit to an elderly patient only a few weeks earlier, she herself had climbed that path to that very back door. She felt first winded, and then stupid for not having pieced this together before. The book that had been so instrumental to her medical vocation was about *her valley, her patients*.

The following lunchtime at work, the doctor mentioned her discovery to the older partner, who confirmed it and filled in the details. That handsome house with the blue paintwork and tall chimneys across the valley from her own: that was where Sassall had lived. The modest stone building, now a private house, on a spit of land between two lanes: that had been his surgery, although, of course, he had visited patients all over the valley. She also now learned of Dr John's tragic postscript. Her own edition of Berger's book predated the death, so she'd had no idea how the story ended. Now the winded feeling redoubled at the thought that from her own doorstep she'd been looking across to where the 'fortunate man' had died in such awful circumstances.

Yet over the months that followed, it came to be his life's work and not his death that occupied her thoughts. The privilege of working, albeit for only part of the week, at his former practice sealed something in her mind. Surely the sheer synchronicity of it presented an opportunity, the chance to develop and to modernize his legacy of longitudinal medicine, based on relationships, and within a community she had already grown to love. Her older colleague, Dr John's former partner, was not far off retirement, so she discreetly made her aspirations known, at length extricating herself from her other job, and in January 2007, she became a full-time partner at the practice.

Today, the doctor's softly uttered yet steely conviction that she will remain here for the rest of her working life speaks not of any dearth of ambition, but rather the audacity of it. In a world of modern medicine, where many patients feel they rarely see the same GP twice, she has become, and intends to remain, a pivotal figure in this valley. It is, perhaps, the payoff of her teenage wager with herself, or the golden thread that connects the remarkable Dr John to the world he left behind.

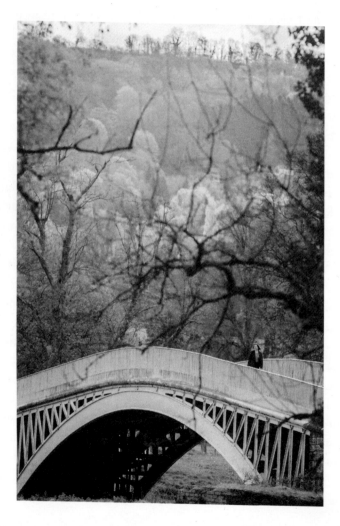

III

IT WOULDN'T BE like him, but she wondered for a moment whether the man had been drinking, as they walked together up the corridor from the waiting room. It wasn't that he smelt of booze, as patients did from time to time, that stale, chemical sweetness rising from the pores, or the sprightly cocktail of white wine and mouthwash she caught on the breath of a well-dressed widow at the end of yesterday's surgery. But no, the doctor consciously pulled a draught of the corridor air between them into her nostrils and could detect nothing other than the smell of wood shavings, a few of which still clung to the man's overalls, and a trace of carbolic soap that reminded her of school. His gait, she noted, was as steady and strong as ever for a man in his sixties. There was no hint of the confident sloppiness nor the studied deliberation of someone three sheets to the wind. Yet there was something odd, slurred, about his speech. She asked him about the house he was working on with his son, just up the lane from the primary school: a new extension wasn't it, when did he think the build would be finished, 'I hope Gareth's doing most of the ladder work', et cetera. His replies were terse and factual as usual, but each utterance today was accompanied by an unruly whistling from between the back of his tongue and his molars. He sounded as if he had a boiled sweet in his mouth.

Once seated in the consulting room, she smiled and focused on him, as if there were all the time in the world, as if there were not four patients waiting and she, the doctor, running late again. She never could bring herself to cut a consultation short in the name of brute efficiency.

'So how can I help today?'

The doctor has come to favour this opening gambit over any reference to what might be 'wrong', 'worrying' or 'seems to be the trouble'. It feels like a positive, collaborative way to begin, one that puts both doctor and patient on the level, two grown-ups with a task ahead that they can work on together. She likes the way that it both cuts to the chase and yet leaves the subject matter wide open.

'Thing is, doc, I've got toothache. Started maybe ten days or two weeks ago, and there's me thinking it'd settle down, but it hasn't. It's bloody sore now.'

The man lifted one freshly scrubbed hand to his jaw-line. 'Pardon my French,' he said. She made a small wince of empathic concern. She's learned that mirroring a patient's demeanour or idiom is useful for re-establishing rapport, even with a patient she knows well. Always something of a social chameleon, at ease with patients of all backgrounds thanks to the odd blend of working class and smart equestrian in her childhood, mirroring comes naturally to her.

Toothache can be miserable, she said, and asked the man whether he'd been to his dentist.

'Well, no.'

He paused, clearly hoping she'd step in, but she let the space breathe, so he continued.

'So I was thinking some painkillers and antibiotics would do it. Think that's all I need. Had a look in the bathroom mirror and I can't see anything. Just hurts. Tooth looks OK.'

He enunciated 'tooth' not with an 'oo', but an 'uh'. Tuth. It's a common pronunciation around the valley, but today it seemed to create the illusion of distance between the man and his offending molar. She asked whether he had tried for an emergency appointment. Again he shook his head.

'Thing is, doc, I can't see a dentist. I just can't.'

Apologizing, she explained that GPs these days are not indemnified to undertake any dental work. She could prescribe painkillers, but really if it came to antibiotics, this was dentists' work. I'm sorry, she said.

'I'm not going to sue you, doc. You know that. And I don't want to be a nuisance. You know I hardly ever come here. But I can't go to the dentist. Full stop. Haven't seen a dentist in more than fifty years.'

Astonished, she asked how he'd managed, what he'd been doing about his teeth all that time. They'd never before had occasion to discuss it.

'If they get really bad, I just take them out myself. I've done that for years.'

She tried and failed to master the expression on her face.

'Pliers,' he said, as if to set her mind at rest.

The man cocked his head back a little, and pulling on a pair of medical gloves, she wheeled forward on the chair to look into his open mouth. He watched her face, as she gently held one cheek and pulled the other out to get a clear view of what resembled the surface of a strange planet, craters and outcrops in alien groupings, a hint of infection on his breath.

'I know I haven't looked after my teeth as I should,' he said, as she peeled off the gloves, 'but you've got to remember when I was a boy, wartime rationing on sweets had just ended. Early '53, I think that was, so all of us kids had gone for it. It was Bev's dad used to have the little sweet shop up on the corner there. Anyway, we had this travelling school dentist, terrible man, did the rounds at all the village schools. Struck off in the end, I think. But what he'd do was he'd get you in his chair, and he'd do a trench job. Drill and fill. Four teeth at a time.

Then he'd claim for four fillings.' The man's hands had visibly tightened on the arms of the chair. 'So that's why. And don't tell me dentists have changed and that they can drug you so you don't care, because that doesn't change anything as far as I'm concerned. I can't and won't go to the dentist, end of story.'

The doctor thought of her own mother, notably robust, unfazed by anything much, but a confirmed dentophobe, thanks to her 1960s village dentist. If this patient had numerous times chosen the pliers over the comfortable high-street option in the local town, she knew no amount of persuasion, certainly none she could achieve in a single appointment, would change his mind. So there followed in her own a lightning-quick, almost subconscious calculus of risk.

These are the intellectual acrobatics performed by general practitioners dozens of times a day. Invisible to the patient – who merely sees the smile, the nod, the careful attentiveness – a complex cerebral exercise is unfolding behind the scenes. This involves sifting and ranking the range of possible outcomes, balancing one risk against another, from petty to dire, then feeding into the equation the patient's medical and personal history, their stated wishes and likely individual behaviours (which may not be identical), before finally determining the best course of action. In the early years of being a doctor, this feels like having two heads, but with time and experience, the algorithm smooths and speeds up to become more intuitive. Which is not to say that the doctor won't sometimes wake in the small hours and worry whether she got the calculation right. That is the nature of the job.

For the man with toothache, she now wrote a prescription and urged him to return if the pain continued, to which he grinned and shook his head.

'Bloody tuth. I'll let you get on.'

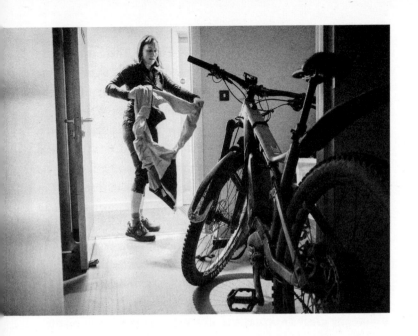

THE MORNING WEARS ON. There's a small girl who decides it's
the doctor's turn for a sticker, pressing a grinning green taran-
tula to her lapel, where it inadvertently remains until lunchtime.
There's a young mother with post-natal depression and wracked
with guilt at shrieking 'What have you done?' at her four-year-
old after he'd tipped poster paint over his baby sister. There's
an aged beekeeper who apologizes for bringing her a urine
specimen in an old honey jar – 'I haven't got a pot to piss in,
doctor' – and there's a middle-aged woman concerned her sister
is taking advantage of their elderly mother's chequebook who
wants the doctor to intervene. There's a mechanic with chronic
nerve pain after an accident years ago, whose reactive depression is filling his head with mortal thoughts: 'I'm in pain three
hundred and forty-five days a year and the other twenty are
unbearable.' There's a dedicated smoker, who cheerfully refuses
to be nudged towards nicotine patches, and a fourteen-year-old

girl having sex with a much older boyfriend: 'I can't believe he's going out with me. I'm so lucky.' Finally, there is an octogenarian widower who cannot cope without his wife and sits opposite the doctor with tears in his eyes: 'I can't even wash the bed sheets without getting them dirty on the floor. What a fool.'

Some days the doctor feels that she is suspended between the old world and an unfathomable future. Of all medical specialisms, indeed of all professions, there can be few others in which one is afforded such privileged access to lives that, in aggregate, span beyond two centuries. Her oldest patient's now frail heart began to beat in the aftermath of the First World War. Her youngest's (if you discount the numerous lives in utero) will likely do so well into the twenty-second century. All those heartbeats. All that experience. All those stories. All that change. There is something both magnificently grand about it, like the great sweep of the valley gorge, and yet miniature, exquisite, like one of the forget-me-nots that sprout between the paving slabs outside her cottage.

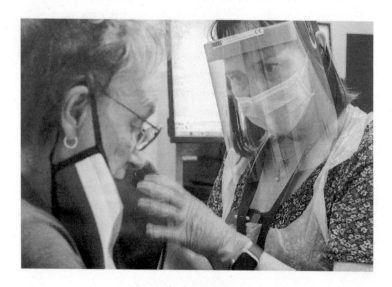

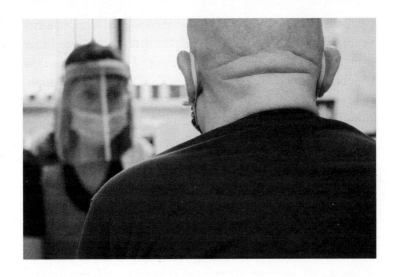

IN SPITE OF a strong continuity of identity, this country practice has led a nomadic existence. The old village surgeries moved about. One decade, the ailing of the parish would present at the cottage between the wheelwright's workshop and the coffin-maker, the next at the lean-to behind the new telephone exchange; then it was opposite the village stores, now long closed; then a converted pigsty down the road. In the old days, here and in rural communities all over the country, a doctor's consulting room was often the front room of his own house. Indeed, it was a mark of Dr John's modernity that he had moved the practice outside the family home, and encouraged his patients to come to him, rather than the other way around. Even so, a significant proportion of consultations remained home visits well into the 1980s and surgery consultations were all walk-ins, no appointment required.

Those days were long gone, of course, by the turn of the millennium when she arrived in the valley, the young doctor with her husband-to-be. By then, the practice had more than twice the patients it had in Dr John's day, and the large majority of consultations took place by appointment only in one of the two surgeries. The surgery to the west of the river was now housed in a building previously home to the authorities responsible for the miraculous advent of mains water in the district in the 1950s. Tucked between the old smithy and a Methodist chapel, this shoebox of a building, so unassuming and yet so focal to basic services here, was much loved by the community. To this day, people still call it either 'The Old Water Works' or 'The Doctor's' (depending on their age), although the surgery itself has long since moved to an angular modern building, with a roof like an open book, on the outskirts of the village. The local press announced its opening in 2012 with liberal use of the words 'state of the art' and reference to its aspirational £1.1 million price tag. The other practice surgery, its twin to the east of the river in Dr John's old village, is the dowdier country cousin, a single-storey modern block that resembles a squashed house, with a playground and fields beyond. While many patients profess fealty to one surgery or the other, in line with whichever side of the river they call home, the practice team – two or three doctors and locums, a handful of practice nurses and healthcare assistants, receptionists, dispensers and administrative staff – all divide their time between the two surgeries, according to the demands of the moment. They are, in their way, as nomadic as their predecessors.

Spend any time trying to wrap your head around the various permutations of building and location, time and place, west of the river or east, and you begin to realize that the real fabric of this country practice comes not from the bricks and mortar at all. It comes from the complex of human relationships within: the camaraderie and collaboration between working colleagues, the rapport between practice staff and patients, the chat between neighbours in the waiting room, which some days sounds more like a coffee morning than a medical setting, and at the centre of it all, that two-way relationship between doctor and patient. Each of these interactions is necessarily pragmatic, current, but they also have deep roots that over time intertwine the individual with the collective, the present with the past. Indeed, it's not uncommon to hear recollections of the old doctors, six or seven of them, stretching back past Dr John, nearly a hundred years. They are part of the warp and weft of this practice, regardless of how medicine and the NHS have moved on.

Around the time that they moved to the new building, the practice did away with the one remaining open surgery on a Friday evening. This had been an ordeal for everyone, a queue of walk-in patients snaking out of the door, often waiting for hours on end and disgruntled if a particularly sick-looking neighbour was called forward before them. The doctor meanwhile would find her head spinning after twenty-three consecutive patients, and when she found herself looking up the dosage for paracetamol she knew it had to stop. One of the locums had already refused to work these walk-in surgeries – 'this is absolutely insane, no one does this anymore' – and in the end the doctor bowed to the twenty-first century. It was undoubtedly the right thing to do, but the consternation within the community was evident. A decade on, they've forgiven her, more or less, but even now patients who've clearly forgotten the hours of waiting will mention from time to time that they preferred the old days and those lovely, relaxed no-appointment surgeries.

This vein of nostalgia for the days of healthcare past is something every doctor has to deal with. Yet it carries a particular piquancy here, because of the longevity of her relationship with many of her patients, and because her career spans the change. She has learned to laugh off the grumbles, or talk them through. Sometimes she'll point out that she's experienced first-hand how the treatment of chronic illness, which accounts for around half of GP appointments nationally, has improved beyond recognition even in twenty years. When she first started here, she'd be rushing with furosemide to people gasping for breath in the throes of acute heart failure; now their condition is better managed with close monitoring and the appropriate combination of tablets. 'Lots of awful things that used to happen, now happen less, so progress brings change, I guess.' That's the kind of thing she says, in that mild but direct way of hers. What she doesn't say is that not all doctors' work is like those midweek hospital dramas on TV. It's not all heroics. Over time she's come to understand that a lot of it unfolds in conversation. Moreover, when you practise in a branch of medicine in which success is so often measured by an absence – the stroke that didn't happen, the heart attack that never struck, the kidneys that didn't pack up – it's easy for people to forget that your work saves lives.

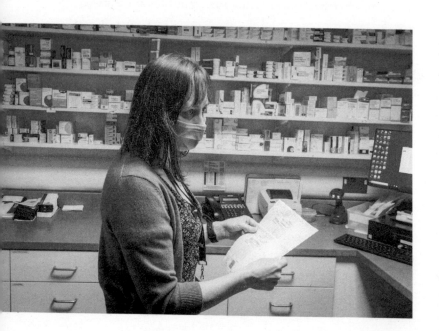

SHE GREETS HIM by his first name.

'Hi,' he replies with hers. 'How's your mum?'

His face looks grey, the colour of white underwear that's been through a dark wash.

Mum's fine, she says.

'And the tractor? You sort it in the end?'

She nods, thanks him, mentions the new fan belt she and her husband fitted at the weekend with the help of YouTube. But the doctor wants to get on with the consultation. She spotted the presenting complaint two hours ago on her appointment list. It made her stomach clench, like someone yanking a drawstring bag tightly shut. Next to his name: 'ceching up blood'. Her first thought was, *That's not how you spell 'keck', how do you spell 'keck'?* She'd look it up later. More pressing was the fact that male agricultural workers in their mid-thirties don't often darken her door, and when they do, it's not for nothing. She tried several times to call ahead, but his phone just rang and rang.

She's known this man since his late teens, knows the whole family. They run one of the few dairy farms round here to have survived the precipitous decline in milk production. In the 1960s, there were dozens of milk producers around the valley area; now you could count them on the fingers of one hand. A few years back, the family were forced to sell the venerable farmhouse that looked for all the world as if its solidity could withstand any shock modern life might throw at it. A software consultant and his pregnant wife live there now. But the man's family managed to retain the land and their herd, now commuting to the fields and the milking shed from a couple of new-builds on the edge of a nearby town. He and his girlfriend live in one, the old farmer and his wife in the other. The landlord at the village pub lets them park their tractor in the car park out back.

I did try to call you, she said. A couple of times. You've been coughing up blood, is that right?

'Sorry, we were milking and there's the suckler herd to feed. I didn't hear my phone, but yeah, I just kecked up a drop of blood, so thought I'd best check with you an' that.'

She asks if he has any discomfort in his chest.

He shakes his head.

Any shortness of breath?

'Don't think so.'

Now that the doctor is sitting opposite him, the light from the window behind her falling on his face, she can see tiny beads of sweat above his dark brows. Not a man who relishes prolonged eye contact, he picks awkwardly at a wisp of hay on his sleeve and, realizing too late it would be improper to drop it on the doctor's floor, he's now stuck with it, pinched between finger and thumb. She can't yet pinpoint a clinical reason why, but, knowing him as she does, he doesn't look right. Something about the colour of his face. It gives her an unmistakable feeling of disquiet that experience has taught her never to ignore.

'Don't mind the dog,' he says, as his collie begins to bark from the back of the Land Rover in the car park outside.

She starts to run through a series of checks: temperature, breathing rate, oxygen saturation, blood pressure. Everything is normal. His lungs are clear. His heart sounds as it should. The only sign of anything out of the ordinary is a fractional elevation in his heart rate, 88 where she'd expect it to be around 70 or so for a man of his age and fitness, but that's not much.

She asks how long he's been coughing up blood.

'I don't know. A day or two?'

No pain in your calves?

He shakes his head.

No recent long journeys?

He laughs. 'Nope.'

This puts the doctor in a quandary. What she is worried about, what all GPs in this situation are very, very keen not to miss, is a blood clot, a deep vein thrombosis in the leg, part of which has broken off and travelled upwards towards the heart. The body's tiniest blood vessels are those most likely to stop the clot in its tracks, in other words, in the brain, where it may cause a stroke, or in the lungs, where it causes pulmonary embolism. In blocking the passage of blood through the lung, the clot starves a portion of the lung of oxygen, causing it to die, which makes the sufferer cough up blood, and in time become short of breath. Untreated, the outcome could not be more stark: acute respiratory failure deprives the heart of oxygen, and without oxygen, the heart stops, cardiac arrest. While the risk of pulmonary embolism increases with age, it is by no means a condition exclusive to the elderly. Furthermore, genetic predisposition plays its part. The doctor knows there's a history of deep vein thrombosis on his mother's side of the family. She and his mum talked about it in this very room only a few years ago, discussing the need for blood thinners after knee surgery.

Then again, a host of more trivial ailments can also cause a patient to cough up blood: a sore throat, a chest infection, gum disease, a nosebleed when blood's been swallowed, even a stomach ulcer. You certainly don't send a man into hospital for a heart rate of 88 and a trace of pink in his spittle, not without inviting derision from the admitting doctor, which she now pictures in Technicolor. And yet that deep sense of unease, that look he has about him, has her considering whether she can somehow concoct a story that will meet the criteria for admission, so that he can be properly checked over. That's how worried she is.

All this flows through the doctor's mind. She thinks of the older doctor when she first arrived here, Dr John's former partner. 'Don't forget,' he'd say, 'disease doesn't always present as the textbooks say. Often it plays its cards in the wrong order. That's why continuity of care, that longitudinal, generational knowledge, is so important. That's what makes you think *Hang on a minute*, when those cards are played out of sequence.' For a moment, the surface of her mind is like the river in spate, churning with jacks and kings and queens and aces.

Some characterize the nature of 'gut feelings' on the part of primary care practitioners as a sixth sense, a kind of clairvoyance on the part of the doctor. Others favour the more earthbound view that gut feelings are triggered by an unconscious process of pattern recognition across a complex array of verbal and non-verbal cues. In this model, a subliminal recognition of correlation with certain medical conditions overrides more conscious thinking about causation, the order in which those cards are played. Indeed, there's now an established branch of medical research, in the UK and across Europe, working to determine a theoretical framework by which to understand the functioning and efficacy of gut instinct in general practice. A recent study of the role of intuition in the diagnosis of cancer offers compelling evidence of its utility, while acknowledging that scepticism on the part of some hospital specialists discourages GPs from citing gut feelings in referral letters. What's unequivocal, however, is that a combination of clinical experience, years in the saddle as a doctor, and continuity of care, knowledge of that particular patient over time, has a significant bearing on the accuracy of a doctor's gut feeling. It's about familiarity with the collective and also with the individual.

Now the man is pulling his fleece back on. There's nothing more she can investigate here in the surgery. She's told him she can't seem to find very much wrong. But look, she adds, I'm worried about you. She says his name. I'm wondering whether we need to get you checked at the hospital. Something doesn't seem right, she says. This drop of blood you mentioned, what did it look like?

'I can show you, if you want,' he says. 'Do you want to see it?'

The man leans down, reaching into the plastic bag he brought with him. From beside a copy of the local paper and a packet of biscuits, he produces a yoghurt pot with a makeshift lid of crumpled tin foil. He peels it back and holds the pot out. The doctor has seen some blood-flecked handkerchiefs in her time, but never anything like this. The pot is one of those with two compartments, one for the yoghurt, one for the fruity topping. Both compartments are full of what looks like cranberry sauce, but is in fact a significant quantity of blood-stained sputum and a number of large clots.

She dials straight through to reception and asks them to call 999. The man is reluctant, but she's already done it.

'You sure?' he says, using her name again. 'You said all my stats were fine. Maybe some antibiotics or cough medicine would sort it. Told Dad I'd be back milking in half an hour. Or maybe I can just drive down there at the end of the day.'

This is one of those occasions when the doctor is firm. No antibiotics, no cough medicine, no going back to work, no driving yourself to hospital. She walks up the corridor with him to an empty side room, puts a hand on his shoulder, tells him to shout out if he feels at all unwell. He can wait there for the ambulance. Won't be long. She'll keep popping her head in.

That evening, the doctor is working at home when she checks the hospital results online. The man is stable, but a scan has revealed significant bilateral pulmonary emboli, that is to say, large clots, both lungs. It was a close call. She looks out into the night as the shadows of trees stir in the wind. For a moment, she can hear the sound of the man's collie barking from the back of the car outside the surgery.

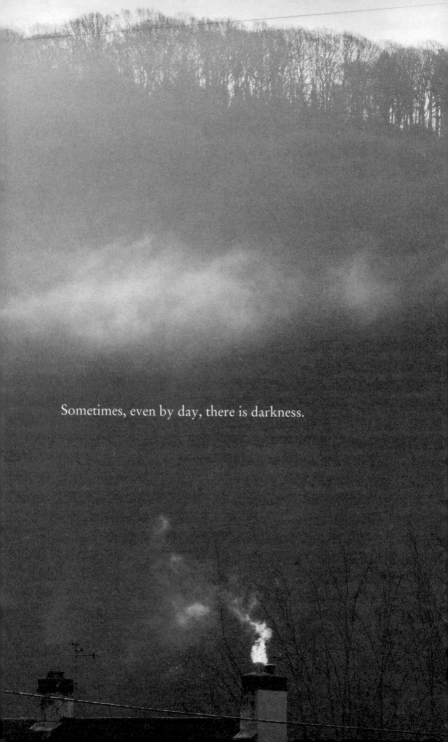

Sometimes, even by day, there is darkness.

This story feels upsetting even now, though it happened years ago, early on in my career. A man who was living on his own. I'd done morning surgery and then there's the list of home visits. One of them was to this man. I didn't know anything about him. He hardly ever saw the doctor and the list just said 'abdominal pain', so for no good reason, I thought I'd go to him first. Found the house. Knocked on the door. No answer, so I did my usual 'It's the doctor, just me.' Opened the door and looked in.

There's a corridor with a kitchen at the end of it and a sitting-room door, then there's the stairs in front. And there he was, legs suspended above the stairs. I imagine he asked for the home visit so that the doctor found him and not anyone who cared about him. I hope that's it, not that he hoped the doctor would come sooner. You have these thoughts.

So I ran in and I got underneath him, and I tried to lift him up to see if I could take the pressure off his neck, but I was too weak. So I pushed past him and went up the stairs and was frantically trying to undo the knot. I'd done some climbing but I'm not brilliant at knots, and there was this feeling, I can't describe it, just I'm hopeless, I can't undo this knot, and it's my fault I'm so useless at knots. *So I pushed past him again, ran downstairs. Found the kitchen. Found the kitchen knives. Ran upstairs again. Push past these legs. Sawing and sawing and sawing and sawing but it was a blunt knife. In the end, I went and found his phone and called 999. I never did get him down.*

I guess what I'm trying to explain is that sense of utter uselessness and failure. Just like I'm worthless. I'm not cut out for this job, *you know? I felt very young and very hopeless. Then the police came, and the paramedics, and I left. I never saw him cut down. Went straight onto the next two visits. Came back, straight into evening surgery, didn't see my colleagues, went home and didn't ever really talk about it. That'd never happen* these days. We'd talk about it now. It would be a 'Significant Event', but we didn't do 'Significant Event Analysis' back then. So professionally, it ended there, when I walked away from the house. I just had a look back through my diaries and I didn't even write it down. My husband doesn't remember it. I guess there's a chance I didn't mention it, I don't know.

That was my first suicide.

The thing is my dad's father hanged himself and he was found by my dad's brother. I never knew my grandfather, but that cast a big shadow over my father's family, and I knew what an impact it had on my favourite uncle. So I suppose I'm glad this man called me. I'm glad no one in his family found him, because, whatever burden it placed on me, it's not the same as what happened to my uncle. Dad never said much about it, but he did say 'That was very hard for your uncle.' You know, just those words. I'm sure every other doctor would have their own horror, but hanging I find very difficult. I've attended several, all uniquely distressing, and that sense of absolute uselessness is just horrible. As doctors, we want to be useful, we're used to being useful, you know? Even if somebody's dying, I can usually make that pathway a bit easier. There's nothing quite like the failure of a suicide, is there? You have utterly failed.

I think that's what comes back to me, and it's absolutely lucid, whenever I see patients where there's a fear of suicidal intent.

IN THE COURSE OF several months of conversation about the doctor's life and work in the valley, the subject of suicide crops up on several occasions. It feels surprising in a woman otherwise so clearly wired for optimism. There are eight specific deaths by suicide to which she alludes through some fragment of back-story, a glimpse of the aftermath, the unanswerable questions or irreparable sadness left behind. It's tempting at first to put this down to some dark shadow cast by Dr John's final deed, or by the grandfather she never knew. But that is to forget the nature of a general practitioner's work in a place like this. She is, after all, the first point of contact, the medical gatekeeper, for every serious crisis of body or mind that arises among her patients. It's a responsibility and a relationship that's come to define her life, and she's built it upon the idea that intense conscientiousness and an active decision to choose hope will always prove useful, however gruelling the circumstances. When that fails, she feels unmoored.

The doctor has, she says, dealt with eleven deaths by suicide in the course of her career, one every two years on average, as well as numerous attempted suicides among patients from their early teens right through to old age. What's more, endeavouring to prevent suicide, to spot the signs and get people help before it's too late, falls firmly within her remit. Patients with suicidal thoughts or a history of self-harm appear in her consulting room every week; sometimes it's every day. Like GPs everywhere, she is more acquainted than most with the complexion of despair.

A study from 2018 suggests that up to 135 people may require support, clinical or pastoral, in the wake of a single death by suicide. For each life lost in this way, the shockwaves spread through family, friends and the wider neighbourhood, and the scars remain for decades. In a community like this one, that grief has a concentration to it that's palpable to their doctor and, over the years, she has realized it is not a sadness she can simply block in the interests of self-preservation. It has to be held with compassion and with presence, and somehow, *somehow*, come evening, it has to be let go.

THE DOCTOR LISTS the things that help her regain her footing when times are tough.

Music (loud).

Exercise (vigorous).

Reading (one novel and one non-fiction on the go at a time).

Nature (in daily wildflower-scented or rain-drenched gulps).

Animals (the horse in the paddock, three adored dogs).

Family (her husband of more than twenty years and two teenage sons, who lately have taken to calling her 'The Mothership'. It is her favourite ever nickname).

For maximum effect, she takes these medicines in combination. They are, in reality, as much a part of her ability to do this job, and keep doing it, as the contents of her doctor's bag or years of training. They make her feel happy, whole, resilient.

None of this is a secret from her patients, some parallel existence to which they are not party. It's hard to hide in a community like this anyway, but she deliberately chooses not to, and people sense this about their doctor. They know her husband, they've seen her boys grow, they ask after them; they see how she spends her time when she's not at the surgery ministering to them. One patient is much amused to hear her warbling along to an Eighties song on her headphones as she tramps up the sodden path at the edge of a stream. Another spots her through the trees one Sunday morning walking with her sons and is astonished to see her stethoscope slung around her neck, as if ready to spring into professional mode at the snap of a twig. As he draws closer, he realizes it's a slingshot round her neck, and they laugh about this as they exchange pleasantries before walking on. The point is she is not simply a service supplier and they service users. Their relationship is not transactional. She is one of them now.

This too makes her feel happy, whole, resilient.

IN THE LAST HALF CENTURY, general practice has seen a more seismic shift in its gender balance than almost any other profession. When *A Fortunate Man* was written, less than a quarter of family doctors were female. Forty years later, in 2007, the very year the young doctor from London became a full-time partner at Dr John's old practice, that figure had risen substantially to 42 per cent. By 2014, the scales had tipped, with female GPs the majority of the workforce for the first time. One year more and General Medical Council data on GPs in training showed that an astonishing 69 per cent of the cohort were women, now outnumbering their male counterparts two to one. There's little doubt that the future of general practice is in female hands.

The doctor attributes this sea change, in part, to the fact that general practice is among the more family-friendly medical specialisms. She herself had always wanted children and this certainly featured in the professional decision-making of her late twenties. Yet she asserts that she's never – not once – felt that being a woman and a mother has held her back. On the contrary, it makes her who she is; it makes her good at the job, she says.

This latter point bears some scrutiny. The main breadwinner in her family, the doctor is quick to emphasize that the arc of her career has been possible because she has always worked full-time, thanks to a husband who paused his work as a recording-studio technician for five years when their sons were born. 'He's my rock,' she says, 'yes, the psychological support, but also in a very practical sense, because he's a brilliant dad. It's not that I was thinking about that when he asked me to marry him. There was no planning in it. I think I just got lucky, but it's life-changing for a professional mother. That was sheer good fortune.'

If you ask her husband, he puts it like this: 'We're a team. We make it work. It always used to be the wife's role, didn't

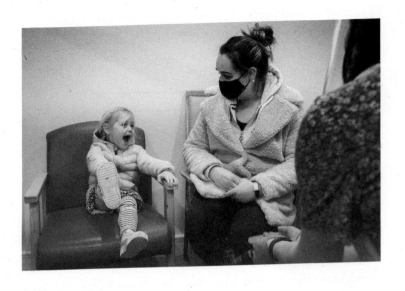

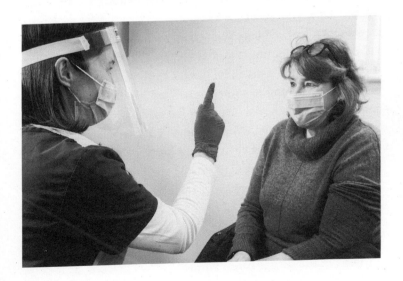

IT WAS ONCE DEEMED to be a village and is marked on the map as such. Not that there's a sign of any sort amid the trees and thick hedgerows. It's quite possible to have lived in this valley for many years and never come across this constellation of squat stone houses set into a patchwork of small fields that conform to feudal boundaries. It is not a place that you ever pass on the way to somewhere else, nor one that you stumble upon, unless you are badly lost in the woods. In which case, you may find it once, but that's no guarantee you would ever find it again. The usual rules of orientation do not apply. Indeed, it has a perplexing, shape-shifting quality about it, this not-quite-village in the trees, as if Escher had abandoned geometry in favour of arboriculture and shaped a leafy place unrecognizable from one angle to another, or one season to the next.

For two decades, the doctor has lived just over a mile away as the crow flies, on the other side of a steep tributary valley that tumbles towards the river from the plateau above. Even so, any time she's called to a home visit across the brook, she seems to get lost. Of late, she's taken to walking with the dogs, rather than attempting the journey by car or the e-bike she favours for many visits these days. On foot, she won't scrape her bumper turning in some constricted capillary of a lane, or come flying off her bike on one of the maze of paths that weave and plunge across the woods. She will arrive sooner, and in a calmer, cleaner state, if she can find her way by trial and error at walking pace. And today, in the dank grey of an autumn afternoon, she is on her way to an elderly lady who has called complaining of shortness of breath.

It's the third wooden gate she has opened in ten minutes, but this, finally, is the right house. She remembers the floral curtains in the sitting-room window, always closed, as if there were many prying eyes in this secluded spot. The woman has heard the gate and opens the door before the doctor reaches it.

'Yes, do come in,' she says, addressing the doctor with title and surname. 'I'm so glad you've come. I've been waiting.' The doctor loops the dog leads over the cast-iron boot scraper under the porch, and, instinctively ducking her head, steps through the low doorway. The house feels damp. The elderly woman quickly shuts the door behind her, and locks it, key and both bolts, top and bottom. The doctor asks if she might wash her hands before they begin and the woman shows her into a cramped kitchen, patting a faded blue towel by the steel sink and tugging closed the curtain in here too. The Formica table in the middle of the room is heaped with papers, letters and documents. The woman sits down at it, as the doctor dries her hands.

Feeling breathless can be very unpleasant, she says, reaching into her backpack for stethoscope, thermometer and oximeter.

'It's been awful,' says the old woman, who looks as she usually does, ancient but robust and pink of cheek. 'Terrible. Like there's not enough air in the world.' The doctor suggests they begin at once with an examination of heart and lungs.

'Oh, I'm not sure we need to do that,' says the woman, 'but what I would like to do is show you a few things here.' She puts on the glasses hanging by a chain around her neck and picks up a sheaf of paperwork balanced on top of a fruit bowl full of small red apples. 'Have one if you'd like,' she says without looking up, and leafing urgently through the papers. 'They're from the tree outside. Now, look at this. It's enough to make anyone ill.'

The woman proceeds to explain, at considerable length, a planning dispute in which she is locked with a new neighbour, recently moved into the house on the other side of her orchard. She produces page after page, letters from her MP, the planning officer, the head of the parish council, builders, architects, plans, maps, deeds.

'It's the worst thing I've ever had to deal with,' the old woman says. 'And it doesn't seem right. Our family has been in this house since the 1930s. You wouldn't know this, because you're new round here too – well, newish – but my late husband's parents were here before we were. My father-in-law worked on the railway that's closed now. He planted that orchard. And then you've got these people coming in from outside like they own the place, and wanting to turn a perfectly good house, a lovely old house, into some great big thing with a glass extension and a carport. A carport! They want to make the most of the view, they say, but why? You can just walk round the house if you want to see the view. And, doctor, it's making me unwell.'

The oblique slopes of the valley are dotted with stone workers' cottages. Many were cobbled into dwellings hundreds of years ago, pigsties or byres upcycled with large rocks from the woods and fashioned into homes, one room thick. Most have their shoulder turned to the prevailing weather, those great storms that blow in off the estuary in winter and push northwards, funnelled by the steep valley walls. Back then, keeping wind and rain out of your house was more important by far than that resolutely modern, central-heating-enabled preoccupation with 'the view'. But in the last fifty years, a certain affluence has blown in with the winds and drifted upstream. Few who would class themselves as workers today can afford these foresters' cottages anymore. Most have been extended, and extended again, the vernacular overlaid with a palimpsest of valley-gazing windows, garden rooms, sun terraces. 'They've grown like potato tubers, our cottages,' says one old-time resident mournfully.

It is this sense of retreat from a simpler past that seems to have pulled the air from the old woman's lungs. On and on she goes. No detail of the planning dispute is too small to explore at length. The doctor humours her. She puts down her equipment on the table and looks at each page passed to her, until she has a lap full of documentation. It takes some considerable time and persuasion on her part to return to the subject of the breathlessness. Reluctantly, the woman consents to the examination, blood pressure, pulse, temperature, oxygen saturation, a good listen to her heart to check for atrial fibrillation, her lungs for infection. And the patient never stops talking.

'I don't think you're going to find anything, doctor. The problem is these new people next door.'

They step into the dark sitting room, so that the woman can lean back on the sofa while the doctor has a feel of her tummy. An abdominal tumour can push up towards the lungs and make a person breathless, but, as they both expect, she can feel nothing out of the ordinary beneath the soft pallor of the woman's skin, nothing other than anxiety, loneliness, indignation.

After three quarters of an hour, the old woman's outrage is spent and the doctor gets up to leave. 'I'm not sure what's to be done,' the woman says, as she unbolts the front door, 'but I wanted you to know, doctor, and I do feel better for telling you about it. Less breathless, I think. Thank you.'

It has grown dark by now. Not realizing she would be here for so long, the doctor didn't think to bring a torch and her phone battery is flat, so she can scarcely make out the path back across the woods. She looks up to the inky sky for the familiar bulk of the hill ahead. Her fingertips touch the rough bark of each tree and the world feels ancient again. One of the dogs picks up a long stick and keeps tapping the back of her calf at irregular intervals. Each time, she starts and looks around. It is a long walk home, the woods velvety black, owls calling, bats flitting between the trees.

THE DOCTOR HAS a particular dislike for the epithet 'the worried well' to refer to patients whose symptoms or concerns don't unfold neatly along pathological lines. To her ear, the term has a casually dismissive air that jars with everything she's learned over the years about the complex layers of relationship that accrete over time. It also carries a nasty tang of 'them and us', those deserving of the doctor's attention and those who, by implication, are wasting her time, as if her time and attention were not the very heart of her obligation to every one of them. In spite of rising use of the phrase by policymakers and some doctors, she's not alone in this view. A recent article in the *British Journal of General Practice* did not mince its words in calling for the 'worried well' label to be dropped altogether, citing reassurance as one of the vital provisions offered by general practitioners to their patients, well, unwell or somewhere in between. This reassurance is not simply a process of going, 'there, there, don't worry, you're not having a heart attack'. It is also underpinned by an understanding that you will be given time to say your piece and that someone will listen, the doctor bearing witness to whatever it is you're going through. The point is that this combination of listening and reassurance is not just a nice-to-have. It banks a data point for future encounters, and more importantly functions as one of the core components of doctor–patient trust. It is kindness; it makes people feel better, and that matters.

Last week, a patient came to see her with his wife. He'd had 'a funny turn', the wife said, 'on Saturday night, a sudden sharp chest pain that made him cry out'. The doctor had examined the man, arranged a chest X-ray and an ECG to be sure, but could find nothing to explain the episode. Perhaps just a musculoskeletal spasm, the doctor said, nothing to worry about. But the wife seemed reluctant to leave the consulting room. It had happened, she said, just as her husband was checking their lottery numbers on the TV, and she'd thought for a split second that they'd won. In that moment, the bungalow and the monotony of retirement had fallen away and she had seen it all: the palm trees, the infinity pool, the jacuzzi, the cocktail in a fancy glass and the vast bed with a tropical flower on the pillow. She'd felt the sultry heat and heard the lilt of foreign guitars. 'We've both worked hard all our lives, and we've never been on a sun holiday, never been abroad, and I just . . . Well, I could see it all, that's the thing.' And back they had walked in silence to the car.

She couldn't quite put her finger on why, but this was one of the saddest stories that the doctor had heard in a long time. The woman hadn't intended to make her feel sad. Quite rightly, she hadn't considered for a second that she might, but what the doctor has discovered over her years in the valley is that a level of emotional engagement with the wider lives of her patients is not only inescapable, but also central to doing the job well.

Another problematic moniker that carries a degree of stigma is the term 'heartsink patient'. Coined in the late 1980s and widely used between doctors, it refers to those whose name on the appointment list gives their doctor that sinking feeling, that *oh no, not them*. It would be a lie to say she'd never experienced it. She has. She's no saint. Yet this is one of those instances when her natural inclination towards introspection has served her well, that tendency to turn every situation over and over and over, until nothing will ease her mind but a long, strenuous stride through the woods.

Enshrined in contemporary general practice is the idea that deliberate reflection on the dynamics of any encounter with a patient, and its correlation to what happened next, is a vital part of maintaining clinical standards. Conducting a contemplative audit of what went right or wrong, and why, is how a good doctor guards against complacency and learns from mistakes.

About ten years into her work here, she was discussing, during an appraisal, a particular patient with a prodigious ability to make her heart sink. She hated to admit it, but this woman was a real pain, combative and uncooperative. She caused a knot of irritation in the doctor's chest any time she appeared in the surgery, which was often. The appraiser had suggested she take a look at some new research into the 'heartsink' phenomenon that might offer another way of looking at this. The doctor did and it was revelatory. Not only did the research suggest it tended to be the less able, less experienced doctors who had a higher proportion of 'heartsink patients' (an excellent nudge to the girl who still wanted to get top marks), but also that the externalizing of this as the patient's problem was fundamentally flawed. Indeed, as the emotional response, that heavy heart, belonged to the doctor, then it was the doctor's responsibility to address it, just as she would if one of her medical instruments was playing up. And in a way, it was. The relationship was playing up and was best fixed not by ignoring the problem, but by facing it, interrogating why you feel as you do about that patient and the responses those feelings provoke, then actively deploying strategies to reframe the feelings and adjust the responses.

This discovery radically changed the doctor's approach to certain troubling or troublesome patients, who no longer rattled her cage in the way they once had, and over time it made her happier in the job. As ever, a diligent and adaptive engagement of both heart and head was required here. Few patients make her heart sink these days.

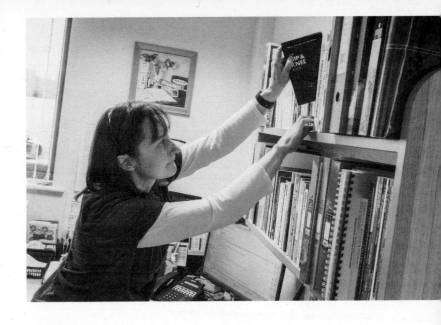

Mᴜᴍ ᴀɴᴅ Dᴀᴅ belong to the old world, says the patient fidgeting in the chair opposite her. They don't understand what life's like for a young person today. They don't understand anything. They certainly don't understand me, the patient says. 'They think I'm ridiculous. They think this is all, like, a fashion or something.'

The doctor knows the young patient's mother and father, not that they have ever discussed this. She suspects they haven't spoken of it to anyone outside the four walls of their house with its neat garden on the smarter of the two estates of new houses at the edge of the village. Everything about their life seems primed to keep the wilderness at bay, right down to the crisp, perpendicular fence that separates their close-cropped lawn from the thick meadow and the trees beyond.

This, their middle child, has always been the 'awkward one' (the parents' words, not the doctor's), given to 'dramas' and 'nonsense'. From what the patient says, she gathers Mum and

Dad are now simply looking the other way, dismissing it as if it's not real, as if there's no such thing. 'Dismissing me,' the middle child tells the doctor, eyes wide.

She's known this patient for the last four or five years, since mid-adolescence. The initial presentation was with acute anxiety and some months were spent discussing a series of problems at school. The teenager never seemed comfortable in that dun-coloured uniform, nor the skin beneath it, which in turn made the mother roll her eyes and suggest a bit of love interest might sort things out. The young patient stopped coming to the doctor with her after that. Now the appointments are solo, straight from the bus after work before going home. Often twitchy and reflexively apologetic, the patient has nevertheless opened up over time. The doctor enjoys these end-of-the-day encounters as the street lights click on outside the surgery. Sometimes the patient appears with brutally short hair and fiddles with it, repeatedly running a palm over the skull-curve of stubble as if to shield it from a bitter wind. The doctor suspects the parents are behind these crew cuts. Other times, the hair grows quite long, and there's something about the way the patient turns that suggests a momentary delight in that feeling of movement above. 'I have always felt that my body doesn't match me,' the patient finally said, out of the blue, during a consultation around a year ago. 'Me as I am on the inside.' The doctor had not consciously entertained this possibility before, but she found herself unsurprised by this non sequitur blurted at the end of an appointment about something else altogether.

Over several meetings following that one, the doctor came to understand that this was a long-standing feeling, one that was there every day of this patient's life. She noticed that the diffidence abated when they were talking about this. 'I've always known,' the patient told her, ever since trying on a cousin's nightie when they were small, although there was always an understanding that this must be hidden from Mum and Dad. It was only through finding support online, months of talking with strangers who'd become friends, that the patient had mustered the courage to mention it to the doctor at all and indeed learned what to say. The day they agreed upon a referral to the Gender Identity Clinic, the young patient asked the doctor if she'd mind a hug. Of course not, she'd said, this must feel huge.

The doctor has several transgender patients, happily living in their chosen sex and taking hormones on prescription. If there are health issues that require sensitive handling – a patient living as a man who needs a smear test, or a woman of many years who would benefit from the test for prostate cancer – then she's found that with honesty and respect these conversations are no different from many confidential discussions that take place in this consulting room. 'It's just about people,' the doctor says.

The waiting time for the clinic in this part of the country is more than two years. Conscious that she may be the only person in the patient's flesh-and-blood world with whom to discuss this, the doctor has followed up with appointments every month or so since the referral was made. It's not enough really, she knows that, but it's all she can do. She wants to keep an eye on the patient's psychological state, coping with this interminable wait, with the decision, with those parents. She lets the patient lead the conversation and, in reality, they talk about all sorts of things in these ten-minute increments of free speech. Pronouns (the shift from 'he/him' to 'they/them' an emotional Rubicon). When to tell their best friend (not yet, they say). Whether it still feels like the right decision (oh yes, yes, yes). And – what they really want to talk about, above all else – clothes and hair and make-up.

'I'm feeling very comfortable today,' they say, smoothing the stripes across their T-shirt and a crease on the thigh of their jeans. 'I've got *my* clothes on. I like these.'

The doctor is not a woman who thinks about fashion much, either on herself or anyone else, so she can see no particular difference from what they usually wear. It doesn't look more feminine to her eye, although her inner voice immediately chimes in – *but what would you know?* There are one or two work dresses in her wardrobe at home that make her feel nice. She saves them for conferences, or days when her spirits are flagging, but as to fine sartorial detail, she's well out of her comfort zone. She says so, apologizes, laughs at being 'hopeless with clothes'.

'And what about eyeshadow? D'you know how to do a fade?'

She hasn't worn eyeshadow since she was at school, she tells them, and she wasn't much good at it then either, but we've got a couple of minutes left, she says, so let's look online.

The consultation ends with a doctor and a patient leaning in to a computer screen, as a make-up artist on the other side of the world paints her eyelids with a palette of iridescence, like cold winter light hitting the surface of an icy river. All three of them are smiling.

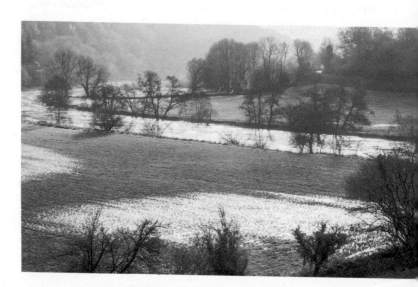

THE RAVELLED WOODLAND that clothes the valley, each ghyll and rocky pulpit, each soft eminence and rolling incline, gives the appearance of having been here since time immemorial, impervious to change. Yet in truth the valley as it is today appears closer to its virgin state than it has in a thousand years. For the woods here have risen and fallen over the centuries, these slopes coppiced, felled, farmed and re-wooded over and over again. Often old photographs of the river, or the long-gone valley railway that used to track the basin of the gorge from one end to the other, show familiar hillsides strangely denuded, as if the forest had succumbed to the clippers of a zealous barber. Still, scattered here and there, a number of ancient trees were sufficiently revered to have eluded the axe. They grow round walls, through fences, on top of rocks, twisting to the invisible arcs of the wind. And so it is that they live on in magnificent, eccentric antiquity amid their young, straight-backed cousins, mute witnesses to centuries of fugitive human lives, sometimes brutally short.

THERE ARE PICTURES of horses on the little girl's bedroom wall. They have been carefully snipped from *PONY* magazine, Blu-tacked in rows, and feature doe-eyed equine faces in pastel harnesses, with captions that say things like 'Pony BFF ♥!!' in candy-coloured fonts. The doctor says how lovely her pictures are, as she finishes examining the little girl in the bed and packs up her bag by the bedside table with its scalloped edge and neatly arranged menagerie of soft toys untouched on top. She asks the girl which horse is her favourite. The child's blue eyes tilt up from the bed, blinking slowly as if her lids were weighted. She looks at the wall for a moment, without turning her head, but she says nothing.

'What d'you think, darling?' says her mother, who's seated at the end of the bed. 'You like that black one there, don't you?

With the turquoise harness. Or what about that gorgeous grey? We love her, don't we? Beautiful eyes.'

'Yes,' says the child, looking at her mother, 'that grey. She was our favourite.'

'We put those pictures up last year,' says her mother to the doctor, as if to explain her daughter's use of the past tense.

The girl is nine years old and has leukaemia. She is under the care of the hospital and has been on intensive chemotherapy for the last two years. She's seen weekly by the child oncologists, but in the last twenty-four hours she's taken a turn for the worse, with extreme fatigue, breathlessness and some swellings in her groin. Before they decide whether she needs to come to hospital, the oncologist has suggested their GP checks for a chest infection or if there's anything simple that might ease the little girl's symptoms. The examination just completed by the doctor suggests sadly not.

It's just the two of them, mother and daughter, in this house on the hill that runs down to the town at the far end of the valley. There are no siblings and the doctor's never seen any sign of the father. She doesn't know why and she doesn't ask. Mother and daughter appear very close, like two halves of a whole. It's rare that the doctor feels she's intruding when she visits patients at home, but she feels it here. Each of them is so focused on the other that she feels as if she is on the other side of a wall made of thick aquarium glass.

The girl now shifts a little and looks at the doctor. She asks her mum for a carton of squash. They listen to the sound of her mother's footsteps retreating downstairs. When she hears the kitchen door close, the girl asks the doctor to look inside the book in the top drawer of her bedside table. She has written a letter, she says, for her mum.

'I thought that Mummy could read it after I've gone,' she says baldly. 'I want to tell her not to worry about everything. I think she'll be upset and I thought it'd help if I write some nice things down.'

There is a pause and the girl adds, 'Because I know what's happening to me.'

The doctor asks if her mum knows about the letter, folding it and slipping the book back into the drawer.

'No,' says the girl quickly, 'and promise me you won't tell her now. I don't think she could bear it now, the thought that I know. That I know I'm dying.'

In the course of her time in the valley, the doctor has come across only a handful of terminally ill children, and never in conversation like this. However, as a medical student considering paediatrics, she did her elective in child oncology, so she knows how extraordinary, how otherworldly, dying children often are. They say and do things that aren't like the things other children say and do. Something about that cruel process, the pain, the fear, the protecting others – 'they become different,' she says. She can't think of another way of putting it.

Now suppressing what feels as involuntary as a reflex to comfort and reassure the child, to say, 'of course you're going to get better, it's going to be OK', the doctor says something that feels futile about everyone doing everything they possibly can to help. You're so calm, she says to the little girl in the bed.

Now they can hear her mother coming back upstairs, so the girl smiles and whispers, 'I think dying makes you grow up quite quickly. But can you just make sure you don't forget to tell her about the letter later on?'

A quarter of a mile back up the road towards the surgery, the doctor pulls into a layby next to a stand of huge, gnarled chestnut trees. They must be many hundreds of years old, and yet still green shoots appear along each of their limbs. She switches off the ignition and stares out of the windscreen.

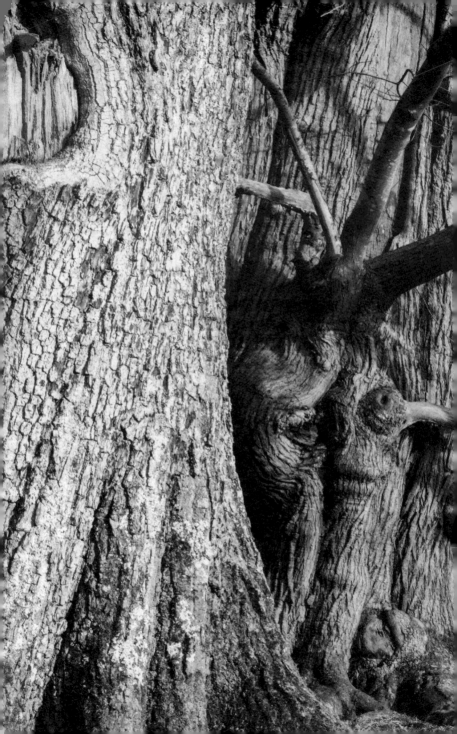

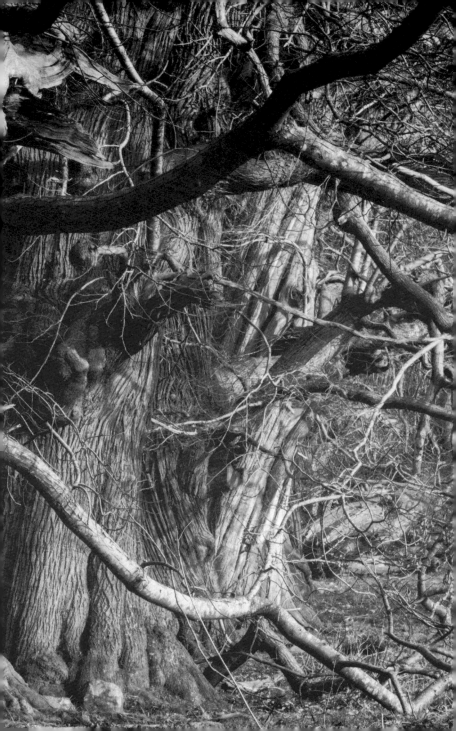

THE VALLEY DOCTOR'S MORNING begins at six. Clean teeth, half an hour on the cross trainer while reading the news on her tablet, shower, coffee, cereal, make sandwiches for lunch, cups of tea for the boys and a hug, leave 7:40, cycle to work, car if it's raining, there before eight. Kettle on, quick chit-chat with the team, then straight into checking the overnight blood results, making appointments for further investigation, delegating what she can to the nurses, reviewing hospital letters, a quick glance at the morning appointment list, and the day's consultations begin.

There's no such thing as a typical surgery, not really, but here is a morning from a few weeks before she will begin her twentieth year as a doctor at the valley practice. It is late 2019.

9 a.m. Middle-aged man, depression.

9:10 a.m. Young man, chest pains, urinary symptoms.

9:20 a.m. Older man, cancelled operation due to anxiety, discussion re. future plan/risks of no surgery.

9:30 a.m. Older woman, gastroenteritis since returning from holiday in India.

9:40 a.m. Middle-aged woman, accidental pregnancy, significant family commitments (frail mother, teenage children), feels continuing with pregnancy impossible, but wants to. Devastated.

9:50 a.m. Middle-aged woman, neck pain, acid reflux, anxiety.

10 a.m. Older man, high blood pressure, prostate problems.

10:10 a.m. Middle-aged woman, severe chest infection, neck pains.

10:40 a.m. Middle-aged woman, right-sided neuralgia, headache, strong anxiety re. brain tumour.

10:50 a.m. Older woman, occasional weakness in legs, difficulty walking, patient not sure why. Examination normal.

11 a.m. Young man, anger management, debts, recent prison, threatening behaviour in surgery.

11:20 a.m. Middle-aged woman, HRT no longer available, anxious re. this.

11:30 a.m. Young woman, anxiety, depression, multiple life stresses.

11:40 a.m. Middle-aged man, infected cyst, excess alcohol, referred for liver scan.

11:50 a.m. Older woman, anxiety, depression, hopes this is reason for memory problems.

12 p.m. Older woman, COPD review.

Home visits:
   Older man, shortness of breath and faintness.
   Older woman, fallen downstairs, refusing hospital.
   Older man, unable to stand up.

The list above tells you everything and nothing about that November morning. It can offer some hint of the range, pace and sheer open-endedness of the work, perhaps. But of what unfolded in human terms behind the fluorescent glow of the surgery windows, of that, it's reductive at best. It's like looking at the receipt for someone's shopping in the hope of conjuring the taste of the meal they cooked, what they discussed as they ate and with whom, the stories they shared. The list might just as easily read: Simon, Danny, Robert, Christine, Sarah, Amanda, Neville, Joanne, Claire, Beryl, Andy, Ruth, Chantal, Richard, Pat, Eleanor, Edward, Jackie, Ron. Or any other list of names. As it turns out, among these nineteen patients, all of whom she sees face to face, there is one cancer, one serious mental disorder, one suspicion of historic abuse, one new diagnosis of heart disease and two onsets of dementia for which the morning's presentations are the first clue. Although of course the doctor couldn't know any of this for certain that morning. It is an intrinsic part of the medical generalist's work that any suspicion of a serious condition is always provisional, never a full diagnosis, always the first staging post on the way to a specialist somewhere else. What she could know was that here were glimpses of nineteen very different life stories, and beyond them, a hinterland of many more lives around the valley that would feel the impact of what she and her patients discussed that morning, as the last few leaves of the year spun in the wind outside.

And of course, the day is only half done. Come mid-afternoon, the doctor's doing paperwork again, making follow-up calls to patients, then preparing for evening surgery and another ten consultations. Twelve hours or more after she's left home, she returns to the cottage on the hillside. There's a meal, a walk in the woods or an hour of TV with the family and another hour and a half at her desk most nights, maybe some yoga, definitely some reading, lights out at 11:30. Sleep.

The doctor has had in the region of 130,000 patient encounters during these first twenty years in the valley. But she has come to understand that the numerical and the technical, even the overtly clinical, is only a fraction of her story here. What lies behind many of these 130,000 encounters is something that so many doctors no longer enjoy: a significant number of high-quality, long-standing relationships that provide the foundation for those pillars of good healthcare, trust, rapport and empathy. While there are friends and neighbours among their number, it's important to understand that these are not friendships per se. On the contrary, they represent a distinct and unique form of relationship, one that is by definition in flux and predicated upon a delicate balancing act of intimacy and distance.

All this has come about partly by design and partly by accident, a confluence of cause and effect in which these things came together for the fortunate woman. Certainly she chose first this valley, then chose this practice, and over time she's learned to work in the way that she does. But it's a small, rural practice not by design, but because this is a small, rural place. That means the doctor is not sharing a patient list of up to 50,000 with a dozen other doctors and seeing forty, fifty, even sixty patients a day, as some of her urban colleagues do. Although she's always busy, that is why she's able to sustain the work and give her patients time. She shares with a small, close-knit team a relatively stable patient list, because people in this valley tend to stay put, and once they've got to know their doctor, if they're ill, it's her that they want to see. It's not a magic trick, but at the same time, *it is*.

The rise of evidence-based medicine over her time in the practice has seen remarkable strides in the treatment of disease and improved medical outcomes beyond recognition. It was certainly transformative in the early days for the young doctor to anchor her clinical decisions within an established framework of best practice, informed by the latest science. But what has proved more difficult to measure, in terms of its efficacy, is the value of the doctor–patient relationship within it. Because this is so hard to quantify in cold, hard figures, performance metrics inevitably skew towards incentivizing outcomes that are easier to define in statistical terms, at a population rather than a personal level. While not a bad thing in and of itself, this culture shift towards standardized interventions for common medical conditions has created a cascade of unintended consequences within primary care, many of which have eroded the doctor–patient relationship upon which it was once built.

Workloads have increased. Practices and their teams have got larger. The role of technology has expanded. Part-time working has become the norm. A portion of the press routinely use the issue of part-time working as a stick with which to beat the rising number of female GPs, but in reality, for doctors of either gender, part-time working is often the only way to endure the pressures of the job. All the while, the wholesale management of risk according to standardized guidelines trumps the judgement of individual doctors. Thus by increments the axis has tilted from an emphasis on the patient to an emphasis on disease, from interaction to transaction. Moreover, as patient numbers have risen, access to a doctor, any doctor, has become the overriding priority, and individual relationships find themselves pushed to the margins. Continuity of care remains much talked of, but it's far less often achieved and, because it's so tricky to measure, it doesn't feature in the framework of payment incentives for general practitioners. It is, by any metric, death by a thousand cuts for the doctor–patient relationship, now so distant from Dr Sassall's story in *A Fortunate Man* as to give the book the quality of a melancholy fairy tale from long, long ago.

There is a rising sense within general practice at large that all this presents nothing less than an existential emergency. This concern that something vital is being lost has led to an intensifying research effort to understand, articulate and quantify the value of the human relationships within medical care, before it's too late. Hard evidence is needed in order to drive policy change. Indeed, a growing body of research links seeing the same doctor over time to a number of significant benefits, both clinical and financial. These include closer adherence to medical advice, better uptake of vaccines, reduced use of out-of-hours services, lower referral rates, better retention of doctors, greater patient satisfaction and fewer emergency hospital admissions. There is even, according to two influential papers published in the *British Medical Journal* in 2018 and the *British Journal of General Practice* in 2021, increasingly strong evidence linking continuity of care to lower death rates. Indeed, the longer the relationship between doctor and patient, the lower the mortality rate, 25 per cent lower after fifteen or more years of knowing one another as opposed to just one. The chair of the Royal College of General Practitioners put it like this: 'If relationships were a drug, guideline developers would mandate their use.'

Yet family doctors, like the woman who stands at her back door in the cold valley air, looking out across the fortunate man's old patch, find themselves an endangered species. Little can she know, as 2019 draws to a close, what fresh perils lie ahead, both for her patients and for the profession she loves. As always, her mind is whirring, full of plans. She's working on a grassroots initiative aimed at vulnerable adults and children in the area. She's galvanized, hopeful for the year ahead.

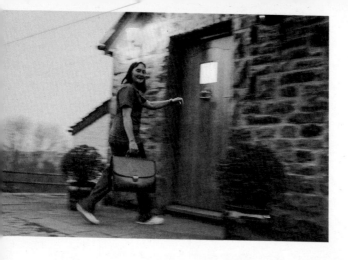

THE RIVER BELOW her house looks to neither future nor past. As it has for countless millennia, it exists in a fast-flowing present and has as many moods as there are days in the year. Sometimes its waters are silent and silvery, sometimes a choral deep green, or, after a storm, a shocking, roaring, blood crimson with soil flushed from the hillside by heavy rain, the current boiling with timber torn from the forest above. Although the depth of the valley makes it impossible in many places to hold both water and sky in one's gaze at the same moment, still the colours of the flow hold the day close, reflecting the heavens' mood in liquid form. This kaleidoscopic virtuosity may be why pretty much everyone who lives round here finds themselves looking to the river as their elder and better, their centre of things. 'Have you seen the river today?' they say to each other when the waters are high, or when they're low, when they're blue, or brown, or clear, or cloudy, mirror calm, or hellfire angry. It is as if their river were an unpredictable but beloved member of the family.

Still, few were prepared for what happened that February, when the river decided to love them back, bursting its banks and pouring into homes from one end of the valley to the other. It was the beginning of what was to be an extraordinary year.

IV

FEBRUARY IN THE VALLEY is hard. For days it's barely got light. The sky is a heavy concrete-grey that weighs upon the high ground, leaving everything below hemmed in, gloomy. It's been raining for weeks, not thrilling, cathartic, thunderous rain, but an attritional falling of cold water from a flat sky, day and night. The river is high and puddle-brown, impervious to what little light there is above, its bulging, furrowed surface like a ploughed field on the move. The ground is waterlogged and dark, any attempt at a walk more an exercise in wading, sinking, sliding through mud. And she can forget about cycling to work, unless the doctor wishes to attend to her patients in the style of some poor Tommy fresh from the Somme. At home, the electric lights blaze all day. Sodden shoes and boots line up on damp newspaper in the hall. Wet coats drip from their pegs, swearing blind they will not dry out before spring, and damp patches spread on the wall where the weather has wheedled its way through the old stonework. The cuckoo-stolen joys of spring in the valley, the meadow sweetness of summer and the majestic glories of autumn are paid for, with interest, in February. Those who live here know this and, for a month, they grit their teeth.

It's a weekend and the doctor is in her study at home, writing a piece about safeguarding for a healthcare website. It's been a punishing week, the floods devastating for a number of her patients who found their homes inundated by the swollen river. They're camping with family or friends now, their sofas in the skip and industrial dryers blowing at their silt-streaked walls. The lower portions of two of the valley villages were evacuated, the local town cut off in three directions and access to the two surgeries limited. As ever in a crisis, her team, at this point all no-nonsense women, came together. Within a heartbeat, they were pooling access to 4x4 vehicles, plotting passable routes and organizing pick-ups and drop-offs, to ensure that the practice was staffed for vital appointments that couldn't wait until the waters subsided.

She often wonders what she would do without these splendid women. Every single day they have the doctor's back. She sometimes worries that she's too busy to demonstrate fully how valuable they are to her and to the practice. An eager proponent of New Year's resolutions, she's made this one of her own for 2020: (1) always try to run on time (she makes and breaks this resolution every year), and (2) make more time for the team.

The website piece she's writing is in the style of a diary, stitched from extracts of her journal. She'll add to it over the coming weeks, whenever a free moment presents itself, but it's hard to know what to write. The theme is supposed to be safeguarding, one of her particular professional interests, but the news is getting in the way. It seems contrary, even parochial, to be writing about safeguarding when so much of the world is talking about the virus that's emerged from China and last week reached British shores. Still, there are only nine UK cases as things stand today, so she attempts, awkwardly, to juggle the two subjects. It is not a fluid pairing.

Early entries say things like: 'February 12th. There doesn't seem to be much in the news about coronavirus. Maybe it will just go away. I'm writing a presentation on adult safeguarding. Primary care is uniquely placed to be a key player in safeguarding adults.' However, as the days pass, it is an impossible editorial line to tread. Safeguarding insights are gradually shouldered from centre stage and the virus takes the floor. 'Doctors' social media groups have been discussing updating wills' (February 22nd). 'Today was the first British death' (February 25th). 'I'm struggling to think much beyond Covid-19. We have only had one patient tested and they were negative' (March 1st).

The doctor has started to wake up at 5 a.m. and stare into the blackness, worrying about what will happen next, how best to keep patients and the practice team safe. She's thinking about stocking up on pasta, in case the family have to quarantine, and finds herself repeating 'Wash your hands everyone!' like a jolly primary-school teacher, although she doesn't feel remotely jolly. 'They're talking about people working from home, closing schools, the elderly self-isolating. It's ridiculous, but it feels hard to know whether this is going to be really serious, or just go away like the Millennium Bug' (March 8th).

A week or so ago, the doctor ordered a new waterproof phone, so that she could listen to music or an audiobook while out in this interminable rain. She can't stay indoors every day, she'll go mad. Yesterday, the phone arrived, and last night she listened to Leonard Cohen's 'Famous Blue Raincoat' in the shower. It helped a bit, but not much. 'Boris Johnson suggested today that we could take Covid-19 on the chin to minimize the economic fallout' (March 9th). 'People I trust are quietly starting to talk about there not being enough ventilators. We have decided not to let anybody with a cough, sore throat or a fever into the waiting room' (March 10th). 'The PPE has been issued. It seems a bit insubstantial, not like the white Hazmat suits you see on the news' (March 11th).

The blog continues for a few days more, but there is no further mention of safeguarding. It's all virus. The daily planning meetings at the practice. The queasy feeling in the pit of her stomach watching tightly packed crowds at one of the biggest horse races of the year. An attempt to see patients under a flimsy gazebo in the car park, foiled by howling winds and hail. The decision from above to abandon face-to-face appointments for anyone with whom a consultation could be achieved by telephone. Their newly fettled treatment room accessed by a rear door at the surgery, where at-risk patients can be seen without contaminating the whole building. The surreal challenges of trying to assess respiratory symptoms by phone, as a teenager reads aloud a portion of a Greek myth and the doctor tries to work out whether he's short of breath. Their lives are changing. She can see that.

The doctor's husband is unconvinced by the light paper mask and plastic goggles she's been using at work, so he's gone to the builders' merchants in town, returning with a full-face respirator mask designed to protect against asbestos fibres and hazardous fumes. She tries it on in the kitchen at home. It looks half disaster-movie, half fancy-dress party; neither, she thinks, will reassure her patients. The sense that everyone's making it up as they go along is vivid and unnerving. She types one last blog entry on March 15th, but her heart's not in it. And after that, she's done. There are other things to be getting on with now.

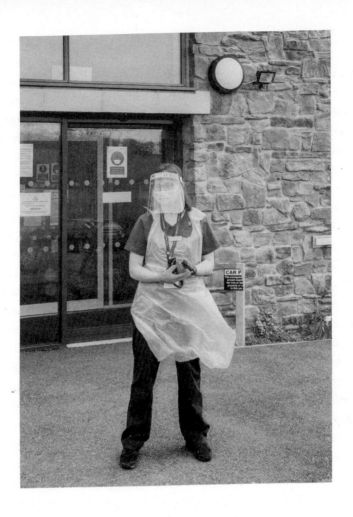

THE DOCTOR FEELS as if two years have passed since writing her diary piece, not two months. The surgery is uncannily quiet, but for the ringing of phones. The waiting room is deserted, yellow and black tape stretched across every other seat. Outside, it is unseasonably hot, the mercury having leapt forward into summer temperatures even before the leaves opened on the trees.

With the onset of the pandemic and the requirement for GPs to don theatre scrubs for all surgeries, the local health board found themselves short. A handful of local ladies sat down at their Singers and set about stitching old bed linen into trousers and tops for the doctors of the county. At first, there were eighteen of the 'Scrubbers', as the seamstresses called themselves; within a fortnight, there were three hundred.

So here she now stands in the consulting room, plastic all over her face, sweltering in a blue swirled duvet cover from the mid-1980s. There's not much dignity in the look, the doctor knows that, but the fabric is soft and strangely comforting as the workload and the deaths mount. It seemed improbable to some at first that the virus would work its way into bucolic places like this, but of course it did. The graphs of infections, deaths and excess deaths here more or less track the national figures. Green trees, blue sky, fresh air, the bubbling curve of a river, none of these, it turns out, is much of a deterrent to a virus.

Trust grows fragile and the doctor feels it. Walking the line between when to encourage acceptance rather than hope for a different outcome is nothing new to her. She's long considered it central to her work here to make these difficult conversations about death and dying a fraction easier, through familiarity, candour, kindness, time. But it's hard discussing by phone rather than face to face something as complex and unfathomable. And now often these conversations are with patients and families she doesn't know. As the hospitals scrambled to empty elderly patients into the community and local care homes, her list is now scattered with new names to which she can put no face, no context, no stories. She works hard at building rapport on phone calls that often last up to an hour, but that's not always enough. This morning, a woman snapped at her, 'You might as well say it. You're just trying to get rid of Mum, because she's old and doesn't matter as much as all the other people.' The doctor explained and soothed her way back from the brink, but it leaves her with a headache. There are another five such calls to make today. Of the death certificates she has signed in the last eight weeks, 80 per cent have been Covid-19 deaths among the frail elderly. This spring is, without question, the hardest time she's ever had to face as a doctor: the fear, sadness and the seething chaos of it, but also the sense that now, more than ever, she cannot drop the ball. She must step up, and step up, and step up. She doesn't even know quite what that means.

Late that afternoon, after several hours on the phone, talking about death and poring over emailed photographs of rashes and moles, verrucae and bunions, she sees her first face-to-face patient of the day. A young mother has brought in her baby boy with an earache. In the ordinary way, such a presentation would be seen by the nurse in the first instance, but the nurse is self-isolating and it's hard to get cover at short notice out here in the sticks. So mother and baby are shown through to the doctor's consulting room. With the migration of antenatal services over the last decade or so to community midwives and health visitors, she doesn't see infants as often as she once did, and she misses it, so the baby boy is a particular treat at the end of an awful week.

One of the hardships of the pandemic is the difficulty of making simple human connections with your patients, through touch, eye contact, gestures, facial expressions. She knows most of them so well that she's got out of the habit of routinely introducing herself at the beginning of every consultation; she hasn't had to do that in years. However, recently she's seen several regular patients while swathed in PPE, and afterwards discovered they hadn't realized they'd seen her at all. For some reason, this felt particularly disquieting. It's why she now opens with a cheery declaration of her name and a 'Hello, it's me under all this rigmarole!' Occasionally, some courtly old gent extends an arm for an elbow-bump and they laugh behind their masks at the strangeness of it all.

Beaming now at the baby boy, as he crooks his sore ear towards a plump shoulder, she's aware that it feels like an exercise in futility, smiling from ear to ear through a mask and face shield. Yet a smile is more than a mouth and teeth – of course it is – because the child's eyes light up and a mighty grin slowly spreads across his face, like a rising sun, a reprieve. As she walks up the corridor after seeing them out, for the first time in weeks, the doctor finds her heart light.

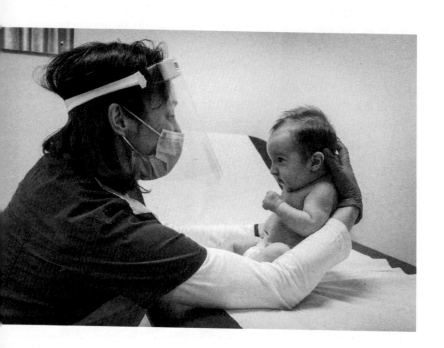

Smiles and eye contact are not, of course, the only non-verbal ingredients of an effective encounter between doctor and patient, the kind that builds a strong relationship. The role of touch is under-represented in medical literature, but is widely agreed to be of significant therapeutical value. It cultivates trust, empathy and cooperation. Furthermore, in moments of distress, fear, pain or bereavement, it plays a vital role in comforting the patient. All this is perhaps not surprising; touch has a role to play in almost all human relationships. What's more interesting is the way in which touch is embedded within doctor–patient interactions, without necessarily drawing attention to itself. She, the doctor, always endeavours to touch a patient in the course of a consultation. It builds bridges, she says. This can be through either so-called 'expressive touch', the spontaneous hand on the shoulder, the light tap on the arm, even the taking of a coat to hang by the door, or through 'procedural touch', the contact that comes from taking a pulse, listening to a chest or performing a physical examination. There is value, she's learned, way beyond what she might discover clinically from the examination itself. Touch matters. It opens doors.

However, this year, she now touches through gloves, on the rare occasions when she touches at all. In a dozen subtle ways, she notices the difference.

How the world has turned in 2020.

The previous incumbent as valley doctor, the one-time partner of Dr John, used to tell comic tales of boundaries breached by patients, sometimes literally: a medical question volleyed through the kitchen window as he was eating Sunday breakfast, or a call to the house concerning constipation at 4 a.m. Much of this ceased with the end of 24-hour care by general practitioners. All the same, the new doctor did find herself, one day early on in her career, seeking refuge under the kitchen table at a knock on the door from someone she knew to be in rude health and likely to disrupt the work she was desperately trying to finish. That day, struck by the absurdity of hiding in her own kitchen, she resolved to be more direct. In the years since, if waylaid by a speculative medical enquiry as she walks the dogs or washes the car, she's learned to say how important it sounds, but that she works better with her computer. 'Why not call in first thing on Monday and we can have a proper chat when I've got your records in front of me and my brain's in gear?' Equally, in certain cases where patients are seriously ill and she holds particular knowledge that might make their management easier at home, she gives them her mobile phone number, and urges them to call her, not the out-of-hours service. This is rarely abused. Generally, she finds patients are respectful of her free time and home space. Few people even lock their doors round here, she says, so a fortress mentality simply wouldn't work.

One day a few years back, she'd nipped home at lunchtime and heard a ruckus in the kitchen downstairs. There she found a patient, her neighbour, bent double, panic-stricken and breathless at the kitchen table, apparently in the grip of a heart attack. She'd reached for the phone to call 999, but he'd waved her off. Finally, when he could speak, it became clear that one of her dogs, in the habit of visiting the neighbours in the hope of a sausage, had eaten some rat poison from the man's garage. The effort of running with the terrier in his arms had nearly finished the neighbour off, but all was well, man and dog intact. It was one of those stories they'd laugh about when the households nearby got together for barbecues on the little green between their houses, or over Christmas morning sherry.

Those days feel a lifetime away now. As the pandemic takes hold, it's hard for the doctor not to feel disconnected from the daily encounters with patients. She finds herself craving the impromptu, the less than vital. The doctor's partner in the practice has been off work for some months and is now shielding, so she is essentially flying solo and carrying a heavier workload than ever before. Most weeks, she has nine or ten surgery sessions. So much, she thinks, for spending more time with the team. In spite of the fact they are under the same roof from dawn till dusk and continue to provide the best support the doctor could imagine, she's running to stand still. They all are.

In the first flush of the crisis, the community rallies, as do communities all over the country, all over the world. Soon a group of villagers have organized medication runs from the surgery to elderly residents isolating at home. The group takes the doctor's first name and calls itself her 'Army'. The name makes her wince, but she's grateful and proud of what they're doing.

As the months wear on, the doctor finds herself doing away almost entirely with her surname and the honorific. This isn't a conscious decision, rather an intuitive one. Perhaps it's connected to the weight names carry when you can't see a face, either through layers of PPE, or because you're on the phone. Perhaps it's simply an attempt to warm up the chilly business of remote consultation, to keep the relationships alive. Some of her team bristle at patients asking for the doctor by her given name, or even worse, by the jaunty diminutive reserved for family and close friends. 'I mean, it's not the pub or a shop, is it?' says one of them. 'You're not going in and asking for a pint or a bag of sweets.' But the doctor doesn't mind. 'I've done it subliminally,' she says. 'I don't think I need that formality. I don't need people to respect me in that old-fashioned way. A consultation is about teamwork, so you want the conversation to feel as comfortable and supportive as it possibly can, but equally if the patient likes a bit of formality and wants to call you Dr So-and-So, then I'll mimic that, I'll fit in.' The doctor has one patient who greets her warmly by the wrong first name altogether, 'and I'd be quite upset if she called me anything else now.'

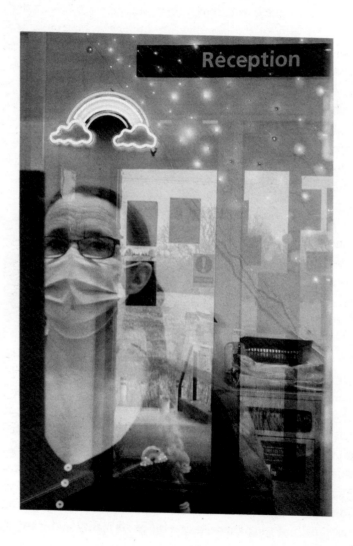

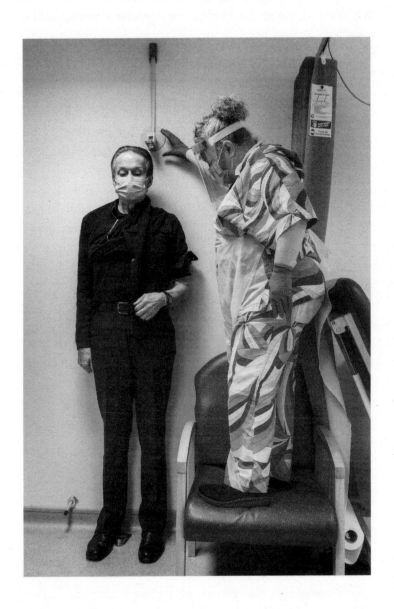

His voice on the phone was light, boyish. He sounded younger than the age on the screen in front of her, and relieved that the doctor was checking on him, although he kept saying sorry for taking up her time, as if this were all somehow his fault. She'd called him the same day his positive test came through, more than a week ago, and every other day since. Just to see how you are, she'd say, check what's going on. He was just glad to speak to anyone, to be honest. His girlfriend was holed up in the lounge downstairs, he said, 'keeping her distance.' Good, said the doctor, well done. She left a microwaved lasagne outside the bedroom door now and then, he said, and sometimes they'd chat for a minute or so, him half tucked behind the door, her out of sight at the bottom of the stairs, but he couldn't really face eating, 'can't even watch the telly.' He'd just been in bed, he said. Half asleep, he said. 'Feeling crap.' High temperature. Shivers, shakes, freezing cold, boiling hot, freezing cold again. 'But I've already told you this,' he said, 'sorry.'

The doctor asked about the cough, was it still there? 'Not really,' he said. What about breathlessness? 'No, breathing's fine,' he said. She asked if he had a book or a newspaper lying around and could read her a paragraph or two, just to check. He mumbled his way through a review of the 2019 Corvette ZR1 from a car magazine by the bed, managing entire sentences about its 'monster-power performance', 'front-mounted V8' and 'optional carbon-fibre spoiler'. 'Just like my car,' he said, deadpan.

This new tool for GPs to test by telephone for breathlessness hardly feels like cutting-edge medicine, but the doctor was satisfied at least that he hadn't stopped mid-sentence to gasp for breath, as a few other patients had, before being shipped off by ambulance.

Make sure you keep drinking, won't you, she said. Loads of fluids. Sounds like you're doing everything you should. I think you're probably turning the corner on this now, but look, I'm just a teeny bit concerned about the rigors, that shivering's been going on for quite a few days. On balance, I'd like to get you in here, double-check you don't need antibiotics. Just to be sure there's no bacterial chest infection there on top of the Covid. What d'you think? Can you manage that?

'No problem, doctor,' he said. He'd need to get dressed, but wouldn't be long. He was only three minutes away on foot, but didn't want to bump into the neighbours – 'they're old, either side of us,' he said – so he'd come in the car.

Half an hour later, a scruffy blue hatchback pulls into the empty car park. He phones through to reception from the car and waits for the doctor to emerge in full battledress. He is a large man in his late thirties, doesn't match his treble voice at all, nor that tiny car. She thanks him for coming in, hands him a face mask, squirts sanitizer into his outstretched palm, and says, Follow me. They make their way past the steps to the main entrance and round towards the rear of the building, through a tall wooden gate to the back yard, past a row of tomato plants in growbags gifted by a grateful patient, past the glass door to the staff kitchen – Nearly there, says the doctor – and they track the wall to a fire door at the back. She notices how slowly he's moving. Three times he pauses, to lean first with his hand on the gatepost, then with his shoulder against the surgery wall. 'Sorry, doctor,' he says. 'Sorry, I'll get a shift on.' The doctor is now convinced there's a chest infection, and is beginning to wonder whether the man may need to go to hospital after all. Perhaps the Covid has exhausted him, or maybe he's dehydrated and his blood pressure is very low. No hurry at all, she says and smiles pointlessly behind her double masks. Try not to touch anything, she adds, once we're inside. Let me get the doors.

The 'Covid Room', as they now call it, has two small windows, each propped open to a grassy bank and thick hedgerow behind. The vanes of the vertical blinds stir in the breeze, throwing prison stripes of weak sunshine across a narrow couch positioned starkly in the centre of the room. Alongside are two plastic chairs and, bolted to the ceiling above, the jointed mechanical limb of a medical examination light. The work surface that runs the length of one wall and used to be filled with medical supplies is now empty but for a slab of disinfectant wipes, two sharps bins and a box of medical gloves. Outside the window, a tiny goldcrest is in full voice, its song like a wheel squeaking on a hospital trolley.

The man slides into one of the plastic chairs and looks at her in all her garb, as she takes his temperature. It's quite high, she says. 'Yeah I don't feel that clever, but you must be roasting dressed up in all that.' Oxygen sats next, she says, then she'll have a listen to his chest and they can work out the best course of action. The doctor slips the sats monitor onto his finger. Normal blood oxygen saturation is between 95% and 100%; anything below that is a cause for concern, below 92% an all-out emergency.

She looks at the reading. It says 58%. Must be wrong. She tries a different finger. 58%. So the doctor gently rubs the man's fingertip with her own gloved fingers to warm it and she tries again. 58%. Think the machine's misbehaving, she says. She tries it on her own finger. 99%. *Shit.*

She read a paper about this some weeks ago. Silent hypoxemia. Some medics call it 'happy hypoxia'. An infernal quirk of Covid-19 observed by frontline doctors in the early weeks of the pandemic, this is technically a medical impossibility, where a patient's blood oxygen plummets (hypoxemia), but with no outward sign of respiratory distress, no breathlessness, no air hunger at all. These are the cases where one minute the patient is chatting to the doctor or reading a magazine, apparently without discomfort; the next minute, they're dead.

An almighty flush of adrenaline washes through her. This man could die on her right here. The goldcrest is still piping at dog-whistle pitch beyond the window and time uncoils into invisible filaments of a second, each stretched to gossamer in her mind.

She fetches the oxygen and slips the mask over his face, murmuring a few soothing words. With studious calm, she asks her colleague on reception to call 999, explains what details to give to the call handler, 58%. Very important that neither colleague nor patient catch a trace of the doctor's fear. It's all under control, everything's fine, we're doing what we do, the ambulance is on its way. The man asks if he needs to fetch anything from home first. No, she says, best to stay put. They've got everything you'll need there.

The man is admitted straight to intensive care, where he remains for several days. In the end, he survives, but the episode haunts the doctor for many weeks. She cannot pass his blue hatchback in the car park without a shudder. Far from being a case where she credits some gut feeling with having saved the day, this is an instance in which the very absence of any real foreboding on her part alarms her profoundly. How could she not have known? What did she miss? She must have overlooked something, some sign, some catch in his breath. She'd had no hard and fast reason for seeing him in person and had very nearly not called him in at all. He'd certainly not merited a home visit in her view and she could have just as easily left him where he was. The man could have gone to bed and died, with his girlfriend watching TV downstairs.

More than once, the doctor listens back to the recording of their last telephone consultation (all calls are recorded for monitoring and training purposes). She puts on her headphones and turns the volume to maximum, fully expecting to hear within the man's account of the Corvette some mortal clue hiding in plain sight, an inhalation or hesitation she'd been too busy, too distracted to notice. That way, at least she'd have something from which to learn, a way to improve, a mistake never to make again. A reminder of her own fallibility would be easier to handle than the Alice-in-Wonderland truth: that if she were to listen to that man recite the virtues of the American supercar again, and again, and again, she would make exactly the same judgement every time.

The doctor doesn't quite know what to do with this knowledge. It nags at her. In the end, her colleagues say, with a degree of exasperation, 'Well, you didn't miss it, did you? He came down here and he's alive.' But who wants a doctor who crosses their fingers and hopes for the best? A cautious doctor, yes, a worried doctor, is a good doctor. And round she goes again.

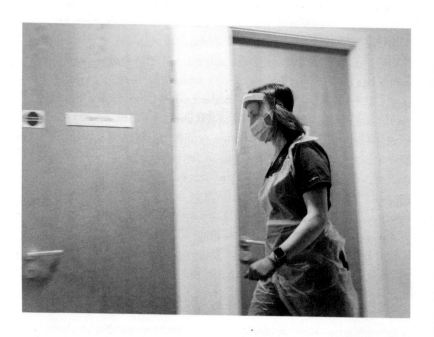

To look skywards in the valley is to read another story about this place. This year, it's the closest anyone gets to an escape. On warm summer evenings, squadrons of swifts wheel about the rooftops of the old houses down by the river, drawing Spirograph circles in the twittering air. At dead of winter, the atmosphere plays tricks, one minute the hillside opposite so sharp and close you could reach out and touch the treetops, the next so distant it becomes a long-ago, half-remembered place. A bright day at the height of autumn sends a wash of light into the canopy, as if a great stained-glass roof had been raised over the forest to protect it from the winter ahead. Or lie on your back in a meadow on a late spring afternoon and the blue above is divided equitably between butterflies that wend past your nose and raptors that carve the updraughts overhead. Usually, far, far beyond, the vectors of passenger planes play high-altitude noughts-and-crosses above it all, but not this year. For many months, the vapour trails have disappeared and the sky has been returned to nature's aeronauts.

For much of the country, the pandemic has been marked by flashing blue lights through the curtains in the small hours, banks of refrigerated units in hospital grounds like grim wedding marquees for the dead, empty streets, boarded-up shops, illuminated motorway gantries telling you to Stay At Home. But here nature seemed to shrug its shoulders, kept calm and carried on. Apart from the missing vapour trails, and the dearth of day trippers in the warmer months, the landscape looks, smells, sounds, feels as it always does, *does* what it always does. Like many valley residents, the doctor finds comfort in this, in knowing that it was all here before and so it will remain, long after the crisis has passed. It sometimes helps to be reminded that you are small, inconsequential.

Where SARS-CoV-2 succeeds in pressing its grimy thumbprint onto the valley is through the absences in people's lives.

No more cinema nights at the village hall, or Pilates With Debs on a Tuesday. No impromptu encounters in the doctor's waiting room or over cider and peanuts at the pub. No Saturday market selling curries and jams, no parent and toddler group at the swings, no Open Mic Comedy or Notable Tree Walks or Weaving With Waste or Ecstatic Awakening Dance. No annual raft race, no spring fayres, no village cricket, no bonfire night, no Santa Fun Run. No pudding club, no book club, no running club, no dropping in or swinging by, or any of the other myriad ways that the people of the valley get together, and which are markedly absent from the photographs in this book, all taken as the pandemic unfolded.

The other absences cut deeper still, of course: families held apart, loved ones lost, bereavements endured. And it turns out that the trees and the sky have a language for this too. Try it. Look up into the branches of a wood, gaze past the leaves and boughs in search of what isn't there, the spaces in between, and you will find yourself drawn into negative space. In winter, an airy mosaic to surpass the finest pavements of the ancient world is laid out above your head: a complex geometry of azure glass or milk-white marble or smoky lead, framed by dark branches. When summer comes and the wood is in full leaf, this mosaic contracts to a firmament of tiny stars, pinpricks of sky in multitudinous constellations that sway and twinkle in the breeze. Summer or winter, this lightscape above our heads is the most subjective of all woodland sceneries, for it resides solely in the eye of the beholder. Shift left or right, tip back, lean in, and the mosaic changes, the stars reconfigure. It is not so different from the human experience of loss: singular, restless, impossible to share, when all you can see is the empty spaces in between.

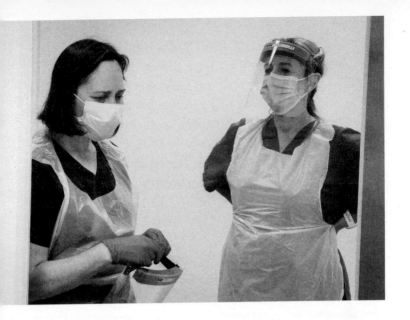

THE ELDERLY MAN was soaked to the skin. His wet clothes clung to his slight frame and made him look even slighter, a little vulnerable, as if he'd been caught out. He'd come to the doctor for a routine appointment to update his medication and check blood pressure. His wife had driven them both, and, in the habit of their long marriage, he had got out of the car to see her back into a tight space in the surgery car park. Thereupon a foul February morning had done its worst. The doctor spotted him out of the window standing there, quite still, watching the car as the rain fell.

'He insisted,' said his wife, laughing as they walked up the corridor to the consulting room, 'even in this shocking weather. I said I could park perfectly well, but you wouldn't take no for an answer, would you?'

The man had smiled and nodded, then shook his head, sending an arc of raindrops from his thin white hair onto the shoulders of his jacket.

Once seated, the doctor asked him how his new blood pressure tablets were settling in. Were they making him dizzy or his ankles swollen? The man was looking at her, but he didn't answer and there was an odd vacancy behind his grey eyes, almost as if she'd addressed him in a language he didn't understand. It flashed across the doctor's mind that he might be having a mini-stroke, but his wife leaned across, gave his knee a gentle shake and her husband was suddenly back in the room.

'I'm sorry,' he said to the doctor, 'it's just that I've always wanted to say *What's Up Doc?* and I was going to today, but I lost my nerve.'

They'd laughed together, the three of them, and the man mimed Bugs Bunny with an invisible carrot. The doctor put it down to the nicest possible eccentricity and thought no more of it. But over the next two years, the man developed Alzheimer's disease and she came to look back on that wet February morning as one of the first signs.

Alzheimer's is caused by a build-up of proteins in and around the cells of the brain, creating obstructions and tangles in the very seat of the self. The disease is hard to identify in its early stages and incurable over time. As months and years pass, the flow of neurotransmitters, the brain's internal signalling system, is disrupted and parts of the brain begin to atrophy. Memory problems and eccentricities extend into judgement, mood and behaviour, vision, language and movement, and ultimately into the most basic of bodily functions. Every disease has its particular cruelty. That of Alzheimer's lies in the way that it sets about dismantling a person and their relationships, taking a human soul apart like a jigsaw, piece by piece. 'It's not him/her, it's the disease,' people will say to husbands, wives, children at the end of their tether caring for someone they love with Alzheimer's, but that offers little comfort, for it is the very essence of the loss.

The man's wife coped with her husband's deteriorating

cognition admirably and for many months. The doctor would see them often during this time and was moved by their dedication to each other. 'I grew up during the war,' said the wife one day, 'so I'm used to getting on with things. There's nothing heroic about it. You just do what you've got to do.' In rare moments of clarity that would blow through like fast-moving weather, her husband would say how grateful he was to her 'for helping me with all those little things', how guilty he felt at the trouble he was causing, 'because she shouldn't have to. I'm ashamed at the work I make for her.'

As the months went by, the wife, who'd always appeared spruce in a practical, plain sort of way, now would fetch up at the surgery looking crumpled and thin, puffy about the eyes, her hair parted flat at the back of her head, as if she'd risen from bed and gone to her labours, without pausing for anything so trivial as a comb. Not given to outward displays of emotion, during one recent appointment, the woman's eyes had filled with tears. The doctor had noticed it with concern.

'She's absolutely exhausted, doctor,' whispered one of their neighbours, who one day followed the doctor to her car outside the village shop. 'You've got to step in. She can't go on much longer like this. I see her hanging out washing four or five times a day. There must be something you can do.'

The doctor understood the coded messages here. She already knew of the incontinence from the patient's wife, and experience told her that this is often the final awful twist of the knife that tips a family from being able to cope with Alzheimer's at home to suddenly not coping at all. She also understood that what this murmured exhortation at the boot of her car on a Saturday afternoon actually meant was 'You've got to get him into care'. Although that was not – nor ever is – her decision to make. She sometimes marvels at people's extravagant ideas as to the extent of a doctor's power.

'Thank you,' she said. 'It's so helpful that you've told me. I can't talk to you at all, of course, because of confidentiality, but you can talk to me. I'm taking it all in and I appreciate it.'

The doctor knows that mental capacity is often misunderstood, both by patients themselves and by well-meaning friends and family. Indeed, that question of whether one has capacity or otherwise is far knottier than many believe. Not only can mental capacity fluctuate from one day to another, even from morning to afternoon, but also, in the eyes of the law, it's decision specific. You may not be capable of one type of decision, but that doesn't mean you're incapable of all decisions. This is a responsibility that the doctor takes very seriously indeed: that she must somehow seek out those islands of capacity on behalf of her patients otherwise adrift on the open sea. If a patient can grasp the nature of a decision, then it is theirs to make, whether wisely or unwisely. Free will is not to be abandoned just because you are unwell. This is key to the dynamics and, perhaps more crucially, the limitations of a doctor's powers of intervention.

In this case, she knows that both the man and his wife wish to remain, for as long as they can, under the same slate roof, in a copse of beech trees at the edge of the village, the home of their fifty-year marriage. Although they are too reserved to spell it out, both of them clearly regard the alternative as the end of the road. Any amount of laundry seems to be worth delaying that, although the doctor cannot help feeling anxious that the wife will make herself ill or have a fall, and then what will happen to her husband? Not that she breathes a word of any of this to the concerned neighbour, hovering at her shoulder outside the shop. Reiterating her thanks, she loads her groceries into the boot of the car and beats a retreat.

It is in the early months of the Covid pandemic that the man has a fall at home and is admitted to hospital with a fractured hip. His wife is not allowed to visit him on the ward and there follows a marked deterioration in his cognition. This is often the case for dementia patients admitted to hospital and acutely so in these terrible days when every rope that anchors them to who they are is cut away. After some weeks, the doctor receives a discharge letter from the hospital. It says that, owing to the man's decreased mobility and the decline in his mental state, he is not safe to return home. Free will ends here. A placement in residential care is arranged, not in the care home by the water-fall at the head of the valley for which his long-time doctor is the GP, but another in a town nearby. The doctor will most likely never see him again.

In normal times – she keeps using this phrase 'normal times' to differentiate from now – she'd have made an appointment for the man's wife to come in. They'd have talked face to face. She'd have passed her the box of tissues on the desk perhaps, held her hand, shown that she understood how hard she had tried and for so long. But these not being 'normal times', she picks up the telephone and she calls.

'I'm only allowed to see him for half an hour once a week,' the wife says, 'through a plastic screen. He doesn't recognize me anymore. Doesn't know who I am. I tell him, but he forgets two seconds later. Doesn't know our daughter either. Someone asked me the other day, nice lady in the village, if I was relieved, and I couldn't think for the life of me what I was supposed to feel relieved about. Because he was safe, she said, but was he unsafe here? I don't know. I'm not sure how to fill the time to be honest, doctor. Found myself watching the television set yesterday afternoon. But I am grateful, so grateful, that they let me go along at all. They're very kind, because they've got all this cleaning to do after I've been and they've got everything else to do as well, so much cleaning. So much cleaning. Yes, it is quite a change, but you get on with it, I suppose.'

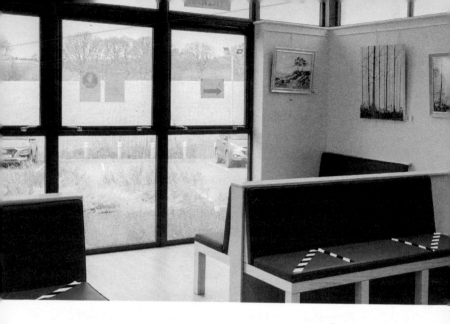

THE CALL TO the wife of the man with Alzheimer's is the first of a morning of remote consultations. The working day began an hour ago, as it always does, with the overnight blood results, hospital letters, and now of course, the positive tests for Covid. Four this morning. She'll call them all. She is the only doctor working today, across both surgeries, so she's in what she calls 'survival mode'.

On the desk beside her there's a pint mug of weak tea. Her love of a strong brew deserted her with the arrival of her children, so she now merely shows the water a teabag and is liberal with the milk. She sips at it, as she dictates the notes from a home visit to a dying patient last night. 'Visit 9pm full stop Sat up in bed alert full stop Blood pressure 142 over 80 comma heart rate 82 comma oxygen sats 94 comma temperature 36.1 full stop Abdomen distended full stop Would usually admit to hospital at this point full stop Patient doesn't want to go to hospital in current climate full stop Realizes that there's treatment to mitigate symptoms in hospital which might not be possible at home full stop Touched on advance care plan full stop Patient prefers not to think about it until a crisis full stop Wife wants what patient wants.'

She started using this software several years back. It shaves a few seconds off the note-taking process, although it always bears some rereading, not least as the program seems to blush in the face of more delicate vocabulary. No problem spelling 'prochlorperazine', but 'anus' is consistently transcribed as 'a nurse', and last week, 'ejaculate' as 'Jacqueline'. She sometimes thinks this tech's most useful role is to make her laugh on a dark day.

Now the phone consultations come thick and fast. She wears a headset wired to a handset-lifter attached to the phone on the desk. Some days it feels like she works in a call centre. This is not how she imagined the life of a country doctor. Those photographs in *A Fortunate Man* of Sassall in corduroy jacket and tie could not feel more remote on days like this, but the doctor turns her mind to what the wife of the Alzheimer's patient said: 'You just do what you've got to do.' She opens the line to the next call and the morning unfolds.

There's a woman concerned about irregular periods, who devotes much of the call to how the supermarket in town has accused her of stockpiling. She has three children of her own and her sister's kids staying. The sister has been living on site at the hospital where she's a cancer care nurse, in order to minimize the risk of carrying the virus to her patients. So now the woman is shopping for a household of eight, she tells the doctor. She buys one trolleyful, sits in the car for half an hour, then goes back to do it all again. 'Couldn't you do me a letter for the supermarket to prove I'm not lying about it?' she says.

There's a young man in low mood, struggling to sleep and feeling paranoid that his girlfriend is 'messing about'. The doctor knows him well, adopts a motherly tone and mentions that the weed he smokes is not helping his mental health. 'How are you even getting it under lockdown?' 'Oh, that's not a problem,' he says, 'cos dealers don't qualify for furlough, you see, so they gotta keep going.'

Next is a call to the doctor's firm ally, the local palliative care nurse, about the man she visited last night. 'He doesn't want to go to hospital. Can you drop in and see them? Wife's exhausted. Hasn't slept a wink.'

And now a discussion with the head nurse at the care home about the advance care plan for a long-standing patient suspected to have suffered a stroke overnight. This is a complicated one, a patient who, long before she went anywhere near the care home, back when her mind was sound, always expressed a profound aversion to hospital. The doctor has known her for the entirety of her twenty years here, making several visits in the early days to the smallholding down a rutted track between two dairy pastures above the valley. Here the woman lived alone with an assortment of bad-tempered animals, a goose that went for the doctor's shins, three or four mangy cats that would claw at her bag, and a donkey that would bray in protest until she was off the property. On each visit, the woman would refuse, in the bluntest of terms, any referral to hospital, whether to investigate suspected bowel cancer symptoms or the sudden loss of vision in one eye. No coaxing enquiry from the doctor as to what would become of the animals if anything were to happen to her made the slightest difference. Her antipathy towards any form of authority, including that of hospital specialists, ran deep. She tolerated the young doctor only because she agreed to home visits, 'wasn't too up herself' and liked animals. But in the end, the whole precarious situation came apart at the seams. Severe memory problems, leg ulcerations, an intervention from social services and a disastrous attempt at care in the home, all led in the end to residential care. There the woman now dwells in a twilight world for which the doctor knows she has no appetite. So she now explains to the nurse the background to the case and the body of documented evidence they hold in support of the woman's wishes not to be admitted to hospital. Yes, she's sure, never been surer of what a patient wants, yes, she'll talk to the social worker.

Mid-morning. The doctor glances at her watch, opens a line and dials at speed. No one picks up. A sigh and she tries again. And again. And again. Someone answers. 'You're terrible at picking up the phone,' she says. 'Now would you please unload and load the dishwasher and hang up the kayaking kit before you do anything else? Dad'll be back mid-afternoon.'

Straight onto the next call and the resumption of the warm, sympathetic tone not always effective with teenage sons, but essential for patients. The patient is a solicitor in her late thirties whose Long Covid symptoms embody the doctor's own darkest fears of catching the virus. These cases make her blood run cold. The woman just about manages to work, but her professional day finishes and she makes straight for bed. She used to do triathlons, but now she can't walk for more than ten minutes without getting out of breath. 'And though you might not notice it, doctor, my brain feels blunt, like thinking's hard work. I can function, but it's a very different life to before.'

Now there are four successive patients with symptoms of anxiety and depression, which loom larger and larger in her appointment list as the year progresses: one man confined to the house with his difficult father, a teenage girl whose parents are so strict about social distancing her boyfriend has finished with her, a woman whose marriage is on the rocks, and an older man who can't bear the loneliness. Two of them say they've had suicidal thoughts. All are first presentations for mental-health symptoms. There is also one cellulitis, one swollen testicle, a new onset of breathlessness, one dizziness, one lower back pain, one rheumatoid arthritis flare, a new patient with high blood pressure and an old one with elbow bursitis. Each of these consultations happens by phone.

The morning ends with a single face-to-face consultation. A mother brings in her six-year-old daughter, the elder of two sisters, the other standing solemn and chastened by the consulting-room door. 'It's my fault really,' says the mother. She was at the computer trying to work, and the girls were upstairs, she says. They'd found the cotton buds and decided to play monsters, shoving two up each nostril, one in each ear and several sticking out of their mouths. 'I heard them roaring, but I didn't realize,' says the mother miserably. The younger of the two had clapped her hands over her sister's ears, shunting one of the buds all the way in, and now the ear was bleeding. One look with her otoscope at the frayed edge where the tympanic membrane should have been and the doctor is making a referral to ENT at the hospital.

'They'll need to pop a new eardrum in there, I'm afraid.'

The mother groans.

'They're banned in our house, cotton buds,' says the doctor. 'I hate them. They cause no end of problems with ears, and not just if you're playing monsters. But d'you know, my husband still loves them. Buys them and hides them in his rucksack. Says "don't tell your mother".'

The morning that began so bleakly ends with two women, two mothers, laughing together, observed by two sombre children.

As THE LEAVES TURN and begin to fall in great blizzards of tumbling gold and red and brown, it becomes clear to the doctor that they are in this for the long haul. Cases of Covid are rising again. There's talk of further lockdowns. Exhaustion, physical and emotional, is setting in. There are more grumbles from patients, nothing serious, but tempers are fraying. The doughty Blitz spirit, which a few months ago saw village ladies don tea dresses to hang VE Day bunting along the hedges in lieu of a street party, has dwindled. The same people now eye with mistrust any unfamiliar face they spot in the lanes, ask questions of what they're doing here, whether it's permitted. Someone posts a picture on the village WhatsApp group of a flashy car, suspiciously clean, that's parked down near the bridge. 'Anyone know whose this is?' There's a succession of admittedly cheerful Saturday flu vaccination clinics – such a blessing to see patients face to face – but the doctor is concerned that the practice team is worn out. Everyone is. Then comes news of the Covid vaccine. It's on its way, it works, an Oxford scientist is on the radio saying 'normal by spring'. A flurry of hope in the doctor's heart is followed almost immediately by a thud of anxiety about logistics, everything that has to happen, and could, between now and then.

She's not sleeping well. She's always said that her years as a junior doctor endowed her with an almost superhuman ability to fall fast asleep in under two minutes and to wake ready to go whenever required. But not now. It's not the morbid dread of the early months of the pandemic. She's become anaesthetized to that. But the doctor knows that, notwithstanding a greater confidence in the efficacy of the PPE, the wider situation remains as worrying as ever. Now she finds that it hits her in gusts, often in the hours when she should be asleep.

Last week, at the end of a thirteen-hour day, she found the single track a mile from home blocked by a fallen tree, its vast trunk green with moss, limbs splayed across the tarmac. Her husband had performed a rescue, installed her in his car, reversed hers back half a mile in the darkness and returned with a chainsaw so they could all get out in the morning, but it leaves her jangled and wakeful. As the clock clicks round from one to two to three, she lies awake listening to the wind stir every tree for miles around. The bowl of the valley amplifies the sound, the hiss of oak and ash by the house joined by a choir hundreds of thousands strong, every dying leaf in full voice. It sounds like the sea. The doctor describes the thoughts that beset her in the small hours as 'earworms', but really the sound belongs to the woods. What vexes her mind is more like the TV news: scrolling clips of crowds cramming onto trains, or queuing on payday at one of the vast budget emporia in the city. I hate it, she thinks, the way this disease is so much worse for people who are not well-off or those who are old and vulnerable. And all around, the woods roar.

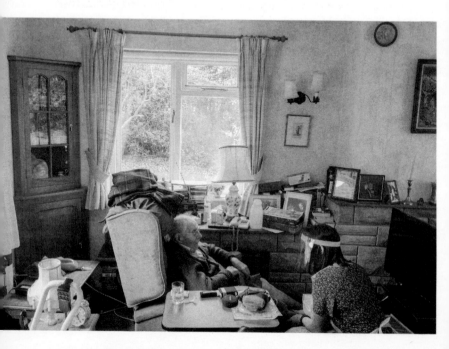

'CAN YOU DIE of a broken heart? I've heard that you can. Is it possible?' The old woman's voice is crisp, precise. She sounds like a radio announcer of yesteryear. Sadness sometimes makes people die, yes, says the doctor, but not always, not by any means. She says the old woman's name. If they were in the same room, now is the moment she would reach for her hand. The doctor certainly knows that for long-standing couples, unions of many decades, the chances of one dying within twelve months of the other are significant. There are instances of heart failure or heart attack. There are people who simply stop looking after themselves, eating enough, seeing people, and whose health declines precipitously. But is it a broken heart? The doctor doesn't know. It's very hard to disentangle and an impossible question to answer of a patient in the first flush of grief.

The doctor has known this couple for twenty years. Initially, she barely saw them at the surgery and didn't realize they were a couple at all. She'd often spot them out walking on the broad forestry tracks above the valley, clearly together, because of the spaniel that would shuttle between them, but one woman always striding several paces in front of the other. She took them for friends, or maybe a pair of ageing sisters given to minor tiffs. But as they grew older and needed the doctor more often, she came to understand that they had lived contentedly together for more than four decades. 'We have never needed anyone else,' one of them said. In recent years, the doctor would visit the house from time to time, on a boggy lane close to the river that would flood on very high tides. She'd learned to sling a pair of wellington boots in the car or leave her biking shoes at the door, if she was called to their house.

By the time the elder of the two women was in her eighties, there were carers who visited once a day, but when the first wave of the pandemic struck, they had cancelled all outside help. The younger and stronger of the pair decided it would be the lesser of two evils if she were to look after the other on her own. Their life was smaller now than it had been, long walks in the woods a thing of the past, but it was still very much worth living, they'd said, of that they were adamant. Having people in from outside simply wasn't a risk worth taking.

Then towards the end of autumn, there was a fall, a broken collarbone and a short spell in hospital for the younger of the two. When she was discharged, such was their relief that the two of them had held hands quietly in the taxi on their way home to the valley. The following day, the hospital called to say that three of the four patients in her bay of the ward had tested positive for Covid and that she should test again. 'We've been so terribly careful, all the way through. We've scarcely left the house,' she'd told the doctor in dismay. 'I can't quite believe this happened in a hospital.'

Now both women tested Covid positive. The younger was symptom-free, but the elder fell ill and, over the weeks, slipped into a highly agitated, delirious state. The doctor's last visit to the house by the river was devastating. There was shouting and confusion, the doctor wrapped in all the PPE she could find, the older woman aggressive and bewildered. In the end, the doctor sent for the ambulance and three days later, miles from her life-long partner, the woman died. The doctor wept when she saw the notification from the hospital. Even after twenty years of doing this, she still feels her stomach somersault every so often and, knowing them so well, this was one of those occasions.

'We had always hoped, she and I, that we'd be out walking and we'd be struck down by lightning at the same time,' says the old woman on the phone. 'But it didn't happen, did it?'

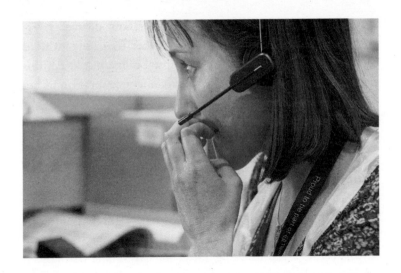

IN THE WEEKS before Christmas, the rate of hospital-contracted Covid-19 accounts for up to 25 per cent of overall infections in the UK. Within primary care, this makes for very, very uneasy medicine indeed. The usual thresholds that would see the doctor sending her patients to hospital have shifted, the lines of risk redrawn. It is not a statistical data set, of course, but consider five recent vulnerable patients, all of whom the doctor would have admitted to hospital in normal times. The three where a decision was made to try and manage their condition palliatively at home are alive; the two admitted to hospital are dead. One of these deaths was thanks to the virus itself, and in neither case was their family able to be at their side.

Such admission decisions are not lightly made, nor one-sided. There is, of course, consultation and sharing of the risk burden with colleagues and the family. But this desperate need to keep vulnerable patients out of hospital is becoming a significant feature of the doctor's clinical decisions during this second wave of the pandemic. Besides, patients of all ages are reluctant to go anywhere near a hospital. In one recent morning

surgery, alongside two patients anxious about delayed refer-
rals and waiting times, there were another six in urgent need
of X-rays or scans who refused hospital point-blank. All this
requires the doctor to perform a dynamic recalibration of her
usual risk parameters. It feels anything but comfortable.

This afternoon, she tries to unwind with a walk before
evening surgery. She needs time alone in the cold, damp air, a
different kind of thinking on your feet. The sky is brewing a
storm, yellow and purple clouds like tobacco smoke in a jazz
club. The land is dark but for a few golden leaves left behind by
autumn, now clinging to the last light of the day, and the river
a smear of sky at the bottom of the valley.

She cannot stop thinking about the care home that lies on
the other side of these woods. There's no Covid there at the
moment, but she's been reading some figures from other residential homes this morning and they have chilled her to the
core. Twenty-five beds, twelve Covid positive. Sixteen beds,
ten Covid positive. A GP in the next county who's tested positive, even though his infection-control processes are watertight.
And there she was, called to see a handful of acutely unwell
patients face to face at the care home on Friday. She's done the
ward round by phone this morning, a Monday, and there are
three patients, not with confirmed Covid symptoms, but out
of sorts, tired, confused. This is how the virus often presents
among the frail elderly. All three are being barrier-nursed in
their rooms as of lunchtime. *But what if? What if? Just weeks
away from vaccination, it would break my heart.* She admits
that her preoccupation with keeping the care home safe verges
on the religious. Sternly, she reminds herself not to over-egg it,
that there's an awful lot more to do than that. And suddenly,
out of nowhere, the sky cracks, an almighty downpour, and,
hood on, the doctor is running for the surgery to dry off before
the first telephone consultation of the evening.

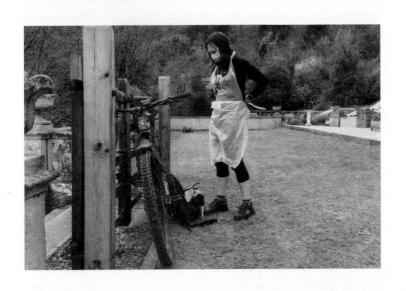

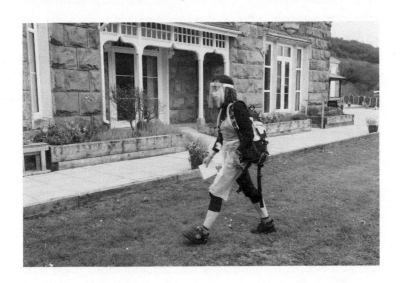

THE DOCTOR'S FATHER was just forty-nine when he was diagnosed with Parkinson's disease and not yet sixty when it saw him into a care home on the banks of the river ten miles and several meanders upstream from his daughter's practice. The disease had wreaked physical and mental havoc in the preceding years, culminating in a garbled decision to leave his wife of three decades. The doctor simply says, 'Bless Dad, it was a mistake. He recognized it was a mistake.' After several years in the residential facility upstream and now in a very frail state, he transferred to the care home for which his daughter was the doctor-in-charge. Another GP agreed to take responsibility for his medical care, but when the doctor finished her ward round, she'd stop with her dad for a spell. He was always to be found in the old sitting room with its high corniced ceiling and grand Victorian sash windows. Together they would look out across the valley treetops, or if the sun was shining, she'd wheel him to the terrace outside to watch the shadows of clouds moving across the slopes below. Just three weeks later, he died.

We hadn't known he was so close to the end when Dad moved there, but his life had been shrinking for a long time. He'd been in the other residential home for eight years and before that he'd been in a little house in town for a year after he left Mum and before that he'd been in their big farm. Each of those moves had resulted in fewer and fewer belongings, less and less. But I'd felt very strongly I wanted his old oak book-case and all the books to come here with him. There was no chance he was ever going to look at those books, of course, but I wanted people to see him as a man who was interested in those things. I put up a few photographs of him too. I was just trying to show them the man he had been, because by then he wasn't really that man anymore. That was the only time I'd spent in that room, not with him there, just putting it all in. So when Dad died, I went straight down there and I had three hours sitting in there with him. It's a lovely room, downstairs in the old part of the building. Beautiful views. I think he died on a Thursday, then I was back in working on the Monday for the ward round and there was somebody new in that room who needed to be seen. That was strange. It felt almost like 'Are you going to be a baby about this or are you going to be able to cope? Of course, you're going to be able to cope.' And so in I went. I don't think it had any impact on my meeting with the new patient, but I must admit it was a destabilizing feeling. Even now, on a ward round I find myself thinking 'There's Dad's room' and it'll always be Dad's room on that bend in the corridor, even though he was only there three weeks. If it's empty, I just pop my head in and have a moment thinking about him, that time sitting with him. It's a big thing losing a parent, isn't it?

The doctor's father had taught her many important things about life: the power of optimism, the value of seizing the day, a deep love of dogs and horses, a sly way at backgammon, the correct volume at which to play Supertramp's 'Dreamer' (very loud), the simple joy of apple slices offered on the tip of a very sharp knife. But above all, it was her father who taught the doctor how to talk to people. He lives on, not only in the bond she feels with the care home, but in every conversation she has as a doctor.

Dad used to listen to what people said, I mean really listen, not wait for a gap in the conversation to say his thing. When there was a pause, he'd feed in a question to keep the conversation going. He explained that you know already what you were going to say. This way, you learn new things. What's funny is that people came away saying, 'That Jim's a nice chap, he's really interesting.' But they didn't know much about him. What they'd enjoyed was his interest in them.

If you were to search for a guiding philosophy behind the

doctor's relationship with her patients – why she loves the work, why she's good at it, why her patients trust and like her – then you need look no further than this. Her father was not a doctor, nor did he know, certainly to begin with, that he was raising one. This was not the stuff of textbooks. This was about being human and how to relate to other humans with warmth and decency.

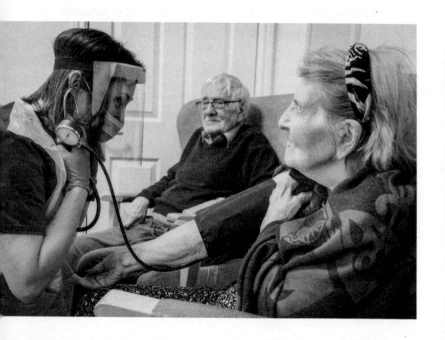

EVERY YEAR, come December, the valley practice does what the doctor calls 'Father Christmassy stuff'. They encourage the community to donate clothes, toys and books to package into age-appropriate Santa sacks for the women's refuge in town or for local families in need. Usually by halfway through Advent, the storeroom behind reception is crammed to the rafters with goodies, but not this year. Infection-control protocols preclude it. In spite of the fact that the practice manager crept round early one morning and festooned each desk, including the doctor's, with tiny fairy lights, Christmas feels sombre this time. A moment of respite comes with a call from one of the doctor's friends. Her children have been having a clear-out and they've found an embarrassment of lovely things, many of which have never even been opened. Would it be useful to anyone? she asks. The doctor has just the person in mind: a single mother, lives in the social housing up by the main road, five kids, three jobs that only barely pay the bills. The doctor texts her immediately. She can see that the message has been picked up, but there's no reply that evening, nor the following morning. She's in agonies, convinced she's caused offence, but at lunchtime, finally, a reply. That would be amazing, the mother says, that'll do Christmas. Thank you, she says, followed by several exclamation marks and a Christmas tree emoji.

It's a small thing, perhaps, but there's something about this that renews the doctor's spirit. The mother is happy. Come Christmas Day, her children will be happy. The family who've offered the gifts feel happy, any prior extravagance expurgated by passing their good fortune on. And the doctor feels happy for putting something simple together in a community she loves. Optimism has been hard in 2020, delusional much of the time, but not hope. Hope is different. She still has plenty of that.

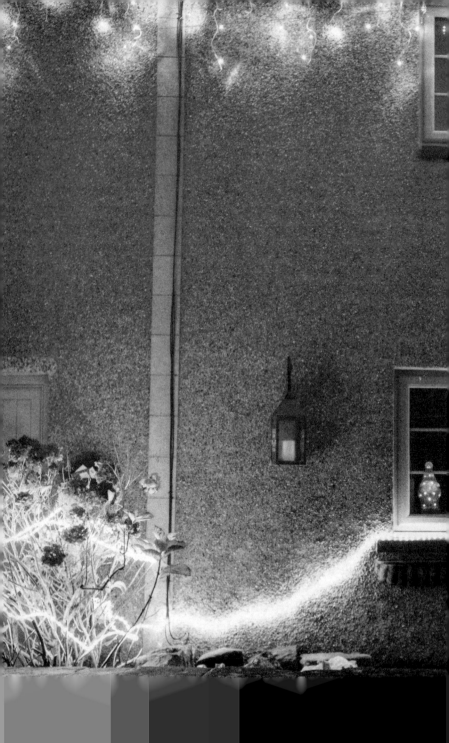

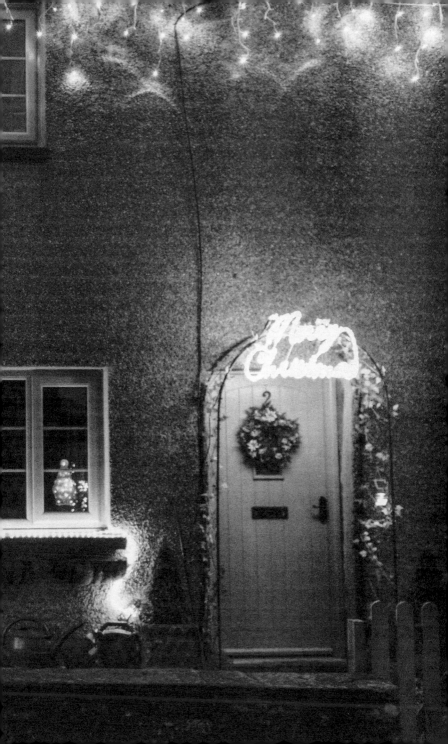

ON CHRISTMAS MORNING, the valley doctor is, at last, not working. She's peeled the vegetables and her husband is busy cooking, so she puts on her headphones, lines up an audiobook, whistles for the dogs and heads out for a walk before lunch. It's a beautiful day, sharp, bright, cold. At the margin of the woods, near the highest reach of the valley, where the tree cover breaks for a patch of damp heathland, she meets a patient also walking her dog.

'Oh, I don't want to disturb you,' says the woman, 'not on Christmas Day. You must relax. Don't stop and chat to me.' But the doctor does. They talk for some minutes about the virus, of course, and the vaccinations that are coming 'soon', says the doctor. She says how the news that the vaccines will be here in the new year is the best Christmas present she can imagine, how it will mean she can get the care home safe, get everyone safe, but the woman stops her.

'You do remind me of old Dr John, you know. Not in your manner, of course. He used to come into the pharmacy where I worked and he'd be ranting and raving and swearing as he did, but it was all forgiven, because his motivation was quite clear. His wife was his absolute anchor, you know. Without her, he was lost. It's funny because my husband and I were talking about this just last week and we said how lucky we are to have had two doctors in our lifetime who loved their patients as much as you do, as much as he did. Someone wrote a book about him. Did you know that?'

And with a 'Merry Christmas' the doctor and the patient part company by the heath.

'THERE ARE SUCH THINGS as national or social crises of such an order that they test all those who live through them,' wrote John Berger in the closing pages of *A Fortunate Man*. 'They are moments of truth in which, not everything, but a great deal is revealed about individuals, classes, institutions, leaders.' Berger was not writing of pandemics of course. His preoccupation was the troubled relationship between the individual, structures of power and the march of history, as he paused to imagine the choices Dr Sassall might make in some future, unspecified Great Upheaval. To the contemporary reader, it's one of the more opaque passages in the book and it's hard to know whether Berger would count Covid-19 as such a crisis or not. All the same, those two sentences seem to echo in the extraordinary events of 2020 and beyond with an uncanny prescience. They read like a warning, or a clarion call, or a lament.

For the doctor, this much was true: yes, the crisis was a test like no other, both for her personally and for her profession; yes, it offered a stark revelation of what matters most in her branch of medicine; and yes, there would be tough choices ahead for them all. For everyone knew by now that simply returning to 'normal times' was no longer an option.

'Covid-19 has produced the biggest change in the organization of UK general practice for 200 years,' wrote the authors of an editorial that appeared in the *British Medical Journal* in late 2020. The pandemic was, they argued, 'a fork in the road for general practice'. While face-to-face consultations had fallen in the early months of the crisis to around 10 per cent of their previous level, the effect of the pandemic on primary care was, at that stage, largely overlooked by policymakers, both at home and abroad. It's significant, for instance, that no practising GPs were included on any committee of the UK's Scientific Advisory Group for Emergencies (SAGE). Although the number of face-to-face consultations increased in the autumn of that year,

V

ONCE IN A BLUE MOON, a fallen tree will right itself, its branches restored to the sky. As the storm passes, the winds change direction, or an obliging human sets a chainsaw to the fallen boughs, some imperceptible shift of balance takes place. Now seeming to baulk at its own quietus, the prone tree creaks into the vertical, its tangled disc of roots filling once more the void it left behind. This is one of an assortment of small miracles with which those who live in the woods are familiar. Tree surgeons know it and take precautions not to be catapulted through the canopy. Parents warn their children never, ever to climb on or behind a recently fallen lime or chestnut, beech or poplar. But no one will deny the thrill that such a thing is possible. It's a rare opportunity to behold not a moment of creation but of deliverance.

Doctors are accustomed to such moments in human form. Much as endings dominate their bread-and-butter work, they are also privy to the wonder of survival. This morning, the doctor is talking on the phone to one such patient, a woman who tells her that last week she celebrated her seventy-sixth birthday with a cake made by her grandchildren and left on the doorstep, as they sang from the other end of the icy garden path.

A year or so before the pandemic, the woman had undergone major surgery for a complicated cancer of the bowel.

Always destined to be a risky operation, both she and her husband knew as much, and a post-surgery bed was set aside for her in intensive care. Everything that could go wrong then did go wrong – kidney failure, liver failure, respiratory failure – and she had lain there in that intensive-care bed not for a few days, but for three months, at the very doors of death. One Friday afternoon, her husband was told her prognosis was so poor that it was time to consider withdrawing life support. He had understood, but was distraught and said that he needed the weekend to digest and discuss it with their children. Come Monday, some unseen shift of biological balance had taken place. To the surprise of her consultant, the woman's condition had not only stabilized but improved. No grim decision was required and soon she was out of intensive care. Six weeks more and, emaciated but alive, the woman came home to their cottage on the ridge that faces outward from the roof of the valley across to the dark mountains in the west.

The doctor heard the details of the ordeal, not from the hospital discharge notes (which made no mention of the potential withdrawal of support and ensuing reprieve), but in a routine follow-up appointment at the surgery. The doctor always tries to do this with patients who've had a long spell in hospital. It helps, she finds, if they can tell their side of the story; there's always something valuable to learn. So it was that the tale had tumbled from them, both husband and wife, as they passed the narrative one to the other and back again.

Within six months, the woman was returned, more or less, to full health. She was as improbable as a fallen tree that one day stands up. Her husband, she told the doctor, liked to call her 'the one that got away'. 'Or Rasputin, when he thinks he's really funny,' the woman said, although the doctor had seen the expression on her husband's face and it wasn't comedic.

When, last November, the woman contracted Covid-19

– she had no idea how, they'd been so careful – both she and her husband braced for the worst. The woman describes it to the doctor this morning on the phone in terms of feeling that there was a finite quantity of second chances of which she had already enjoyed more than her share. She'd spent a week in bed and two weeks more feeling tired and 'off', but there was no hospital, her husband hadn't caught it, and by now, January, she felt her old self again. 'It's strange, but I almost feel guilty,' she says. 'Well, I would, if I didn't feel so lucky. But when I think of . . . well, all manner of people locally, it doesn't seem fair, does it?'

THE PROMISE OF the Covid vaccine seems to offer closure on such uncertainty, the endless roulette as to who will shrug off the virus, who will succumb. But in reality, the vaccine doses themselves take weeks to arrive in the valley. The doctor had expected the practice to receive the first delivery not long into the new year, but the days tick past and a batch of the Oxford/ AstraZeneca vaccine has failed, so there are delays in the supply chain. The practice is besieged by phone calls from patients wanting to know why relatives or friends on the other side of the country have been called for their jabs before people around here. A week into 2021, the second wave of the pandemic is now in full flood and the care home above the valley is one of the last in the county with no Covid cases. It's a situation the doctor knows they may lose any day. She and the practice manager spend consecutive afternoons in meetings, making phone calls and writing emails to try and expedite delivery, but none of it makes any difference. Alongside her frustration, she notices almost a modicum of relief at the realization that however hard they try, there's nothing they can do to speed things along. Living here and practising as she does, there's no harm in a reminder of the limits of one's capacity. At least, that's what the doctor tells herself, although at times it's as if the ghost of Dr John himself were rattling at the window to say, 'Fucking do something.'

She makes a home visit to an elderly patient in the village. He has lived here, above the valley, all of his eighty-three years. Dr John was his doctor, of course, and even the preceding doctor, when he was a very small boy. However, this afternoon, the subject is not physicians of old, but vaccinations of old. It seems to be all she and her patients talk about these days.

The old man lives in a modern bungalow in the main village now, but he tells the doctor how he grew up on the steep lane below the Old Church, a tiny medieval chapel and bell tower now oddly set apart from any settlement and suspended below thick woodland at the northernmost meander of the gorge. It was a long way for a small child to trudge, he said, more than four miles through the woods to the doctor's surgery by the old post office in the village. But trudge he had, aged just five, to play his part in the first mass vaccination in the country's history. The disease was diphtheria, one of the leading causes of death in children during the decade he was born. 'Well worth the long walk,' his mother had told him. 'It took all morning to get here,' he said, 'and then I had an injection, and I walked all the way home again. That's what I remember.'

In the middle of January, an itinerant vaccination team from the health board visits the care home near the waterfall to administer first doses. The doctor permits herself a glance skywards and a murmured 'Yes'. Soon after, both her mother and her practice staff are called as NHS frontline workers for their first jabs at the huge vaccination centre in a city sports stadium twenty miles away. It's strange that after all they've been through, the process itself feels almost bureaucratic. It certainly lacks the poetry and drama one might expect of a moment of redemption, but the relief lies in the *Oh well, that's done* mundanity of it, in the whispered *thank goodness*. For the doctor it is tempered by a twinge of guilt at not yet vaccinating the vulnerable in her own community. 'It's nicer, cleaner somehow,' she says, 'to feel the delight and relief for somebody else rather than for yourself.' All the same, she notices how both teenage sons, who have never mentioned any anxiety about her safety at work, nevertheless hug her tightly the evening of her first jab: 'That's great, Mum.' She realizes they have been carrying something of this.

The practice's first vaccination clinic, at the larger of the two valley surgeries, is scheduled for the second to last Saturday of January and twice weekly for months thereafter. Many hours have been devoted by the doctor, the practice manager and their small team to fine-tuning how to get everyone in and out safely, how to time the appointments in order to maximize through-put, while allowing for consent protocols, logging and cleaning. They begin with eight-minute slots per patient, and reduce it, as they get their eye in, to five. Three of the team administer jabs, five log and steer the patients through the process, more than two hundred each day, before sweeping them out at the back of the building to contemplate the rough green-brown of the wet meadow behind the surgery. Here, as the weeks roll on, they will be met by a chorus of birdsong and the vegetable scent of new grass and wildflowers. But not yet, for this first weekend there is snow on the way.

TALES OF HARD WINTERS abound in the valley. These are the shared stories that define a community, the memories that hold people together. Once, years ago, the surface of the river locked fast in a tessellation of thick ice and stood immobile for several days. When at last the current tugged the frozen pavement loose, the clatter of its passage downstream reverberated to the cloud-scuffed crown of the woods above. 'That were a hell of a din,' remembers one old resident. Another man recalls how the narrow lanes at the top of the valley would fill to the hedge-brim with snowdrifts blown from the fields beyond. His father would use the tractor to scrape a tunnel through the snow, he says. Meanwhile, he and his brother would scamper the length of the ice-bound hedges either side, reaching up to twang the telephone wires overhead. Even today, the wind that whistles across the roof of the valley, like someone trying to elicit a musical note from a bottle, carves deep snow into improbable modernist shapes, so many Henry Moores sculpted in white. The villages up here are often separated on winter days from those near the river, by a distinct, ruler-straight snow line. Up here, you can be digging a path to the car, or abandoning it altogether, while your neighbours a quarter of a mile downhill can still see their garden grass poking through a meagre dusting of icing sugar.

A snowbound day presents a particular set of challenges for the rural doctor. It may mean slithering up the icy lane to the care home on foot, holding on to the overhanging branches for traction. Or a few winters back, there was the two-mile trek in wellies and woolly hat to a patient who on arrival was found tucking into beef Wellington with a nice glass of Bordeaux. 'Doesn't he look better, doctor?' said the wife, who ninety minutes earlier had insisted upon the doctor's urgent attention. The two-mile march back through what was now a blizzard afforded the doctor ample opportunity to review her triage skills.

However, the case that repeats on her whenever snow is forecast is what happened when an odd-jobbing neighbour of hers, the most ardent of fettlers, a wizard with bailing twine and wood, rang the surgery to say that he had 'hurt his hand a bit'. The deep snow had caused all but a handful of patients to cancel their appointments that day and the doctor, whose sons were very young at the time, had stepped out for a couple of hours to join them sledging with their grandmother. The younger of the two had grown cold and they'd tobogganed home for a mug of hot chocolate, when the house phone rang. Two minutes later, she was in the car on her way to the neighbour's smallholding up at the top of the hill. The injury was, she imagined, a nasty cut or perhaps an unfortunate hammer blow. She knew this family eschewed much in the way of medical intervention and avoided the hospital at all costs, so she stopped by the surgery for some bandages, fluids and first-aid essentials. The steep lane up to his cottage was impassable, so the doctor parked in a gateway, shinned over the gate and began to walk up through the snow. The man's workshop, in truth little more than a shed, was at the far end of two paddocks. She noticed first the workshop door ajar, next a trail of blood in the snow leading up through the first paddock, over a five-bar gate and up through the second to their kitchen door. She followed it, quickening her pace, and stepped inside. There he was, ashen on a kitchen chair, his elbow on his knee and a tourniquet of what looked like white surgical tape dangling from the bloody hand held above it. In the palm of his other hand, stretched flat as if he wished to distance himself from its contents, was half a thumb. The doctor said his name and he replied 'pillar drill'.

The man's two adult daughters were milling about the kitchen, shifting from one position to another as if uncertain what to do or where to put themselves. The doctor asked one of them to call 999. In Dr John's day, the necessary surgery might well have been undertaken by him, either at the practice or at the cottage hospital in the forest, but not anymore. The man would be admitted to a large A&E department in the city. All she could do was stabilize him and buy time.

Before reaching for the bandages, the doctor looked closer at the mangled hand. The white tape was not a tourniquet at all, but eight or nine inches of tendon plucked from the man's forearm by the pillar drill. He was clearly in shock, his breathing shallow. The doctor inserted a cannula into the crook of his elbow, attached a tube and glanced about for a hook or shelf from which to hang a bag of saline. In the end, she asked the other daughter to stand next to her father and hold it aloft, while she, the doctor, bandaged his hand. Once the fluids were up, the hand dressed and elevated atop a stack of cushions on the kitchen table, the severed thumb on a wad of gauze nearby, the wait for the ambulance inched by.

In such situations, she will undertake various bits of doctorly business, none of them medically essential, but all part of appearing busy and passing the time. She'll take a pulse, temperature, check blood pressure, adjust dressings, chatting all the while, which in turn reassures the patient and their family that everything possible is being done. Above all, it fills the minutes, when otherwise panic and pain could take hold again.

When she looks back on that snowy afternoon, and any number of patient encounters over her more than twenty years here, she understands that part of what she offers those in her care is time. After all, time is all we've got, not in the efficient, managerial, let's-schedule-a-meeting-don't-be-late sense, nor even solely in terms of extending life and postponing death. Rather, she works in the knowledge that time is the finite axis of our lives and that our experience of it matters. For not every minute of a life carries the same weight. Sometimes weeks, months, years can flit by, light as gossamer, but in pain, fear or distress, just ten minutes can weigh heavy as a year. How you treat people in those minutes makes a difference, the doctor knows. She is here to help carry the heavy time, so that her patients may seek out lighter days again. This is as true for the dying man counting his hours, or the young woman struggling with depression, as it is for a make-do-and-mend man who has severed his own thumb and is waiting for an ambulance in the snow.

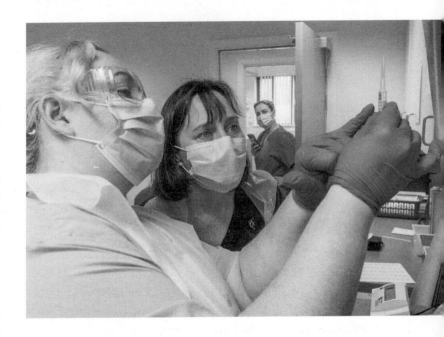

THE FORECAST OF SNOWSTORMS at the first Covid vaccination clinic does not make for an easy night's sleep. This will be the first time in many months that the doctor's most elderly patients have ventured out into their valley. Sacks of salt and grit have been shipped in to the surgery and are stacked by the doors for scattering at first light. Still, the doctor has spent a significant portion of the night worrying that some poor old lady, in the hope of deliverance from the killer virus, will slip in the car park and break her hip. More than once, she climbs out of bed in the small hours and peeks through the bedroom curtains to scan for the dim blue of a night-time snowfall.

But morning comes and, today, nature has been kind. It's bitterly cold and icy, but as yet, no snow.

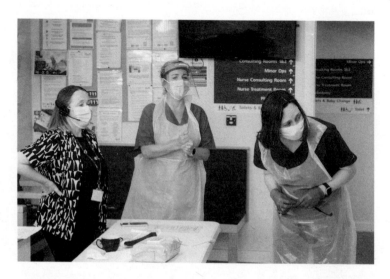

The doctor gets to the surgery early. Everybody in the team is there early. Everything is ready early. The atmosphere among them has a shimmer of electricity. It's quiet, focused. This is it. Before the first patients arrive, there's a lull and the women gather in the empty waiting room, keyed up, like runners before a race. The doctor, not usually given to oratory, finds herself speaking.

'My goodness, you guys,' she says. Her voice is raw with emotion. 'You are, and you have been, unbelievable. Ever since March last year. At no point have I ever asked any of you to do anything, *anything*, and it hasn't been done and you haven't come straight back two minutes later, saying "What else can I do?" You are amazing. Thank you.'

There's a cheer, some tears dabbed, a nose or two blown beneath masks. In her heart, the doctor knows this is not the end of anything, just the beginning of another long, uncertain year. Still, this place, these people, they make her feel hopeful. They are the bedrock of her trusted position in the community; the relationships are theirs as well as hers. Someone lifts a finger to their ear. The rolling crunch of wheels on grit and a tiny grey car creeps into the car park outside the glass doors, a glimpse of silver hair at the wheel. And they're off.

The overt emotion exhibited by the team, all in their forties and fifties, is not replicated in their elders. This is the generation who grew up during the war. There is an occasional misty eye, but mostly what is on display is a matter-of-fact stoicism. There is a festive, galvanized air about the surgery, so glorious to have patients here again, but behind it thrum the lost days, weeks, months, at a time of life when they are in short supply. This has been one stretch of time that the doctor has been powerless to buy back for her patients. 'Good to see you at last, doc,' says an old man, 'I know you've just been on a long cruise,' and he chuckles. One woman presents the doctor with a jar of marmalade. She's complained to the health board about the delays in the vaccine roll-out, but wants the doctor to know the grievance is not with her. 'It's Seville orange,' she says. 'I make it every January.' Another woman comes with her husband, who is sporting a halo of fluffy, white lockdown hair. 'It's good, isn't it?' she says. 'He looks like a dandelion clock.'

Late morning, the doctor notices thick cleats of black mud from somebody's shoes on the floor of her consulting room and scattered down the corridor. She picks a piece up and rolls it between her fingers. It doesn't feel like mud. At the end of the corridor, the practice manager is trying and failing to persuade an elderly lady into a wheelchair to roll back out to her son waiting in the car. The cleats of mud are in fact the rubber soles of the old lady's shoes, unused for nearly a year, which are crumbling and falling off in chunks as she walks. 'No, I won't fall,' she is saying, her voice crystalline in the corridor. 'Thank you, but I don't want a wheelchair. I want to walk.'

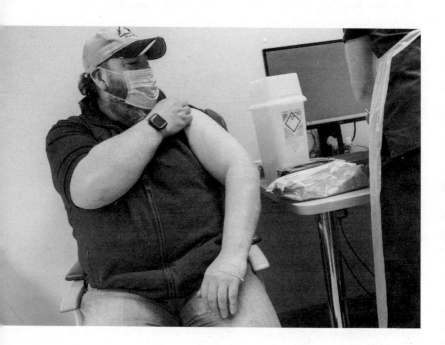

Tucked within a patchwork of small farms on the plateau above the river is an Anglican convent. Home to an enclosed contemplative community nearly a century old, the convent occupies a fine Edwardian building with a chapel, a large vegetable garden, an orchard and sixty acres. Photographs from the 1970s show a vibrant, self-sufficient community of twenty-three nuns, tending to their beehives and chicken coops, milking cows, cutting hay or digging potatoes, making butter, bread and cheese for their modest, silent suppers at long refectory tables, a holy book propped on a stand in front of each plate. Now the community numbers just five professed sisters, two in poor health, a young novice and two more awaiting admission to the noviciate. These days, their provisions arrive thanks to Tesco online and a weekly veg crate from the greengrocer in town.

The doctor is not religious, but there is something about the peace of this place, both atmospheric and metaphysical, that always takes her by surprise. It's quiet and smells of a different age, like a grand old country house, with a hint of polish, damp and old books. It is one of her favourite places in all the valley. Until recently, most of the nuns here were well past retirement age, and she was always struck by the wisdom of these silent old women, another kind of family in which life is sometimes hard. As one by one a handful among them ailed and died, she and one of the more vigorous sisters, now in her early seventies, worked together to tend to them.

'I'm a trained nurse, but not a doctor,' says the nun, 'so I can't diagnose, but the doctor, she helps me, and if I need things, she knows I need them. The way we live, most people don't understand it, but it's very different from a medical point of view if a patient is part of a religious community like ours, because these are not easy places to live.' She talks about the silence, the way it forces you to confront not only your own foibles but other people's. 'And you can't get away,' she says.

'But the doctor, she understands all that. She's interested, a very good listener and very reassuring. She keeps me going, I think, because we've had some fairly heavyweight issues. Just recently, the doctor's got us a Covid vaccine for someone who's come to help with the cooking, as we all live so close together.'

Ask her whether she considers this work spiritual at some level, and if she minds whether the doctor is a Christian or not, and the nun is sharp. 'It doesn't matter to me at all. I don't know about her private life. I know she's got sons and rides bicycles, that's it. But we've heard a lot during the pandemic, haven't we, about how people have learnt to be loving and caring, and I think the doctor was already loving and caring. I don't know if you'd call that spiritual or not. The point is she's a person, not a service. That's why she's always late for appointments. It's because she spent time with the one before you. And, if you ask me, that's a very good thing.'

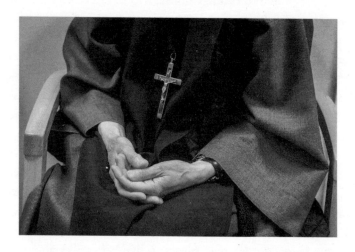

THE NIGHT AFTER the first Covid vaccination clinic, deep snow.

The woods look like a black-and-white photograph as she walks to work on Monday morning, the only colour the red Gore-Tex of her jacket. If she can, the doctor always commutes on foot on a snowy day. Rather than a travel precaution, it's a seasonal treat, a chance to drink in the valley at its loveliest, combined with the fun of crunching your boot-prints into two and a half miles of virgin snow. She'll never be too grown-up for that. She feels the same way about shiny conkers in autumn, which fill the pockets of her coat although her sons have long lost interest in them. And buttercups that glow under your chin. And shouldering past the head-high bracken that crowds the meadow paths in summer. So many childhood delights that have never quite fled, but the best of the bunch is snow. She arrives at the surgery with a pink nose and a smile on her face, in spite of everything that a Monday-morning surgery at the height of a global pandemic may have in store. Ten minutes later, she is an adult again, in a complex world.

AS THE MONTHS have passed, the process of consulting by telephone has grown easier. She's worked hard at it and she's got better. The doctor still misses the nuance of the face-to-face encounter, but she's found, especially with patients she already knows, it's possible to glean a good deal from reading their voice, their pauses, their evasions and emotions. All the same, the last two telephone appointments this morning are ethically delicate. The first is with a teacher at a local primary school, regarding a girl diagnosed last year with autistic spectrum disorder.

The doctor has known the family since she was born, but first discussed this with her parents a year ago, when the girl was struggling at school, and increasingly refusing to go at all.

She was bright as a spark, but found it difficult to settle or do classwork. The clamour of the playground upset her, the roar of the hand dryers in the school lavatory block made any trip to the toilet terrifying. Even the textured plastic of the moulded school chairs made her uncomfortable and agitated. Mindful of the brevity of a ten-minute appointment as opposed to the six hours her teacher spent with her every day, the doctor had, with the permission of the girl's parents, discussed the situation with the school. They talked about some simple non-medical interventions: permission to use the toilet quietly on her own, with paper towels to dry her hands, a wooden chair fetched from the staff dining room instead of the textured plastic. These requests carry more weight coming from a medical professional than from the family, she's found. But in the end, a referral was made to ISCAN (Integrated Service for Children with Additional Needs).

Then came lockdown and the schools closed to all but the children of key workers. The girl's parents were both postal staff, so she continued attending, and here came the revelation. For now there were five or six children, not thirty, in her class, and the building was quiet, the girl settled and began to flourish. Her interactions grew calmer, her schoolwork improved, she was happy to plait her hair and put on her uniform in the morning. Indeed, the child seemed content at school for the first time her parents could remember. All this made the return to the classroom last September, her final year before moving up to the comprehensive in town, the rudest of shocks. Now as well as the throng of children, and the noise, came the litany of rules regarding masks, class bubbles, social distancing. The girl had spiralled downhill until her parents could barely get her out of the door in the morning. It was only when cases of Covid soared again, they told the doctor, and the second lockdown came, not long before Christmas, that there was a similar reprieve for their daughter. Now with the vaccination programme well underway and talk of when schools might reopen on the news, all of them, doctor, parents and teacher, are preoccupied with how to make the next transition less turbulent than the last. Once more, the doctor's work revolves around the passage of time, in this case the child's school days and her future. There is no easy solution and the conversation between doctor and teacher lasts twice as long as the allotted slot. 'You can imagine how her mum and dad feel, can't you?' says the doctor. 'They love her so much and they've been so anxious. Then they've suddenly seen this beautiful blossoming and this is who she could be, who she probably will be as an adult. It's difficult. We need to keep thinking, keep working on this.' They agree to speak again in a fortnight.

The sixteenth and final call of the morning concerns the postscript to one of the doctor's most complex cases of the last few years. As she waits, listening to the rise and fall of the ringing tone, she thanks God she's not dealing with the central crisis of this case through remote consultation. The woman would never have opened up on the phone. As for the idea of her being locked down at home with that handsome, abusive husband of hers, it makes the doctor shudder. That would have been dangerous indeed. For a month or so, two years back, the doctor genuinely feared that the man might snap and do something terrible. When she thinks of him now, his clean-cut good looks, that easy-going confidence, those clothes that spoke of summer holidays in affluent coastal enclaves, she finds her mind's eye homing in on his bright, white teeth.

She'd known the family for several years and liked the man very much at first. He appeared an exemplary father, the ease with which he'd appear at the surgery with one or other of his small sons effortlessly tucked under an arm, no awkwardness in slipping the child's T-shirt over his head so that the doctor could listen to his chest, and to boot, so the doctor thought, coping with a wife who seemed fragile. Her visits to the surgery always brought a whiff of chaos. The boys would wreak havoc in the waiting room, picking up the river pebbles arranged at the base of the pot plants and lobbing them at each other, their mother growing more tense by the moment. Although always expensively dressed, she would often have a smear of lipstick on her teeth or a corner of her blouse untucked, as if she'd left the house in a hurry. Over many months, the woman appeared in the doctor's consulting room complaining of low mood, headaches, dizziness, and above all, chronic pelvic pain. Every possible investigation was undertaken and no cause ever found. The woman often expressed guilt at finding her life so hard, whilst being so materially fortunate. The doctor knew there to be a strong association between undiagnosed pelvic pain and adverse childhood experiences, sexual abuse or current domestic abuse. Along with irritable bowel syndrome or chronic migraine, it's a symptom that can occur when mind and body merge in a somatic firestorm. Yet on reflection, the doctor had plumped for the first cause, a traumatic childhood, as the more probable, given the oh-so-credible husband, and gently, over many ten-minute appointments, she had fished for whether there might be some past experience troubling the patient. She found none.

The day that the whole story poured from the woman, like burning lava, was the day the doctor knew that she too had been played. It was a textbook case of coercive control. Increment by increment, the woman's autonomy had been whittled away, access to housekeeping money or petrol for the car restricted, expensive clothes chosen for her rather than by her, a daily barrage of verbal abuse, unfounded accusations of infidelity followed by further restrictions on her movements, threats of penury and taking the children away if she didn't comply. There were arguments, sometimes physical. She was barged against a door frame, her wrists squeezed until they bruised. And today, her nine-year-old son had rounded on her, she said, swiping at her face with the back of his hand and, in an echo of his father's words, said, 'You're pathetic, Mum. A total waste of space.'

Over the months that followed, the doctor saw the woman often, always explaining the risks both to her and to the children of remaining in such a situation, and some of the ways she might extricate herself safely. In the end, the couple separated, the husband took a job (and a woman) on the other side of the country and the mother's health improved. Often in such cases of suspected domestic abuse, this is the juncture at which a doctor leaves the story. There is no formal mechanism for monitoring how such a patient is coping in the aftermath. The family doctor simply has to hope that they make an appointment, or if they're on medication, as with this patient, that they turn up for their routine six-monthly review.

This morning, the phone rings and rings. The doctor hangs up and tries again. At last, the woman answers. Her doctor smiles, says the woman's name and her own.

'Oh, I'm so glad I've caught you. Now look, how are things?'

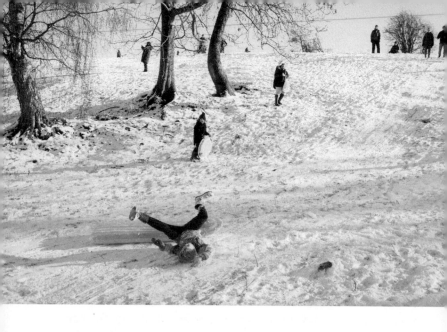

THE WEIGHING OF ethical questions is so central to what the doctor does every day that she relates the process to her capacity for hope. 'What is the right thing to do? How can we, *how can I*, do better?' she says. 'I think we have to just keep trying.' This engagement with the morality of her work, as well as the practical and clinical, underpins every aspect of the doctor's approach to general practice and to her patients here in the valley. There are not always easy answers to these questions, but the key word here is 'practice'. Her life's work is not simply about the application of a body of knowledge to an assortment of human objects. Nor is it the static state of being a qualified doctor who holds that body of knowledge. It is iterative, a virtuous activity in the true Aristotelian sense: a pursuit meaningful in and of itself, both ethically and interpersonally. It is *becoming* rather than *knowing*, and its lifeblood is trust. Looked at in this way, each primary care consultation becomes a waypoint on a journey, rather than a clinical destination at which medic and patient arrive in a timely manner. For a doctor like her, in the fortunate position of caring for many of her patients until the end of their days, the only real point of arrival, in cold materialist terms, is death itself. So the question is can the language of 'medical outcomes' successfully encompass all that will unfold on such a journey, all that quiet calibrating of time? Can its value be measured?

Published in the *British Journal of General Practice* during the second summer of the Covid pandemic, a longitudinal study of continuity of care within general practice in the UK identified a steady and worrying decline between 2012 and 2017. Not only did the percentage of patients who can usually see their preferred GP fall by ten percentage points, so too did the percentage of patients who reported having a preferred GP in the first place (by nine percentage points). In spite of the association between poor continuity of care and poor health outcomes, the failure of policymakers to prioritize continuity has brought about a situation where many patients seem to have given up on the idea of the family doctor altogether. It's natural that people don't much think about the kind of doctor they want until poor health forces them to, so it's unsurprising that younger and healthier patients don't place the same emphasis on seeing a preferred GP. Who cares about this stuff until the moment of crisis? However, another more concerning reason may be that the experience of building a relationship with your doctor, and the trust it fosters, is simply slipping from collective memory. If a good doctor–patient relationship is something you have never known, why on earth would you cherish it, or fight for it? Why would you even consider there to be any alternative to healthcare-as-transaction? This was already the situation before the Covid-19 pandemic, but now as politicians debate remote consultation and digital triage as the default hereafter, that memory of the value of continuity and of the trust built by personal relationships threatens to slip ever further into oblivion.

So if the doctor in this book strikes you as some kind of quaint museum piece, an old-fashioned throwback to an age as gentle and idyllic as the valley in which she lives, then consider why. It is not because her clinical practice is out of date; quite the contrary. It is because, in many places, we have forgotten to expect, or even to want, doctors like her.

The sense of alarm this causes within primary care, ever more urgently since the pandemic struck, has led to calls for a more concerted effort to wrap some hard numerical science around the question. There is a need, some have argued, for randomized controlled trials of continuity in general practice, with a view to quantifying the mechanisms that link continuity to that buzzword of 'better outcomes'. What's needed is something that will demonstrate once and for all that this emphasis on relationships is not simply a warm, fuzzy nice-to-have, but central to effective healthcare, and to the long-term survival in the UK of the National Health Service. The economic imperative here could not be more stark. According to figures from NHS England, general practice provides more than 300 million patient consultations every year, compared to 23 million A&E visits, while a year's worth of GP care per patient costs less than two emergency presentations at hospital. In other words, if general practice fails, as one *BMJ* article put it in May 2021, the whole healthcare system fails.

A medical paper published the same month as the study on the decline of continuity of care proposed not a singular causal link, but an interconnected framework of the mechanisms linking continuity to health outcomes. To the lay reader, what's fascinating about this paper is how obvious it all seems, how any of us who has a relationship with anyone else, personal or professional, intuitively knows this stuff already. Central to the paper is a complex flow diagram of cause and beneficial effect for both doctor and patient. It's hard to do justice in words to its pleasing geometry, but it shows how building a relationship over time fosters familiarity, empathy, understanding, a two-way sense of responsibility, all core ingredients of trust; and that trust then encourages disclosure, improves communication, saves time; which in turn cultivates cooperation and empower-ment, reduces anxiety and mistakes, improves the execution of tasks undertaken together (in this case diagnosis, prescribing, adherence to health advice etc.); all of which adds up in the end to 'better outcomes', reduced hospitalizations, lower costs, lower mortality. It all sounds like good common sense. Yet scientific medicine still has some distance to go in framing this in such a way that health policymakers cannot ignore it.

By way of example, it may seem extraordinary that the concept of 'accumulated knowledge', one of the mechanisms linking continuity of care to better outcomes, was only formally proposed in the academic literature in 1992, a full quarter of a century after *A Fortunate Man* was published. The idea was that treating and communicating with a patient over time accrues a knowledge of that patient, which in turn builds trust, and that this trust then enhances the delivery of good healthcare. Think of the 'accumulated knowledge' of Dr John, from more than three decades tending obsessively to his forest community. Or consider the valley doctor today, and how in so many of the stories in this book, such 'accumulated knowledge' has helped her to identify and understand patients' physical, social and mental vulnerabilities, and to care for each of them as a person, rather than a pathology. Much has been written about the way in which biology and biography entwine in the practice of family medicine. If this can be quantified and framed in terms that mesh with how policy is shaped, then perhaps at last science and story can start working together.

With the stutter of a tractor engine and the crump of tyre-tracked snow, the doctor's husband rolls through the cold, blue stripes of the car park beyond the consulting room blinds. He's here to pick her up, but there's a home visit to do first, so they ride through the monochrome forest, up and over the rise, to a cluster of old brick barns on the side of a steep hill, converted a few years ago into a number of large modern flats. The tractor looks more suited to the yard outside than the neat row of snow-covered cars and ornamental pots of bay, their leaves heavy with fat ovals of white. After the breeze of the drive in the open tractor cab, the cold air now feels motionless, as if nature were holding her breath. Inside Flat 2, a man is dying, not particularly fast. He knows as much. So does his wife. Early on, they would ask, 'How long, do you think, doctor? How long?' But they've stopped asking that now. The local cancer care nurse with whom the doctor works closely said this morning she suspects he may have another five or six weeks left, but she wants the doctor to check on some symptoms of abdominal pain. The curtain at an upper window moves, the doctor waves to the man's wife and pulls on the PPE she's brought in her bag.

The flat is one of those upside-down homes you sometimes get on steep hills. You enter on the first floor, and in this case descend to a modern extension at the back where the bedrooms face an improbably suburban hard-landscaped garden with thick, wild forest beyond.

'That's you, isn't it?' he calls up from the downstairs bedroom, using the diminutive form of her first name. 'I'd know those elephant footsteps anywhere.'

'Yes, sorry, I'll try on tiptoes,' she says. 'Mind if I come down? She's just making tea.'

The doctor is blessed with a heaviness of footfall that belies her slight frame. As a junior doctor on night rounds in coronary care, the nurses used to make her take off her shoes at the top of the corridor to avoid her waking half the ward. As she puts down her bag by the bedroom door, she repeats this anecdote to the grey-faced man sitting up in bed, who laughs and coughs and laughs again. 'And you're only a little thing too,' he says.

At the end of the examination, the doctor sits and chats with the man for a few minutes. He is less anxious than the last time she saw him. He tells her, 'Think I've made my peace with it now, but the wife' – he pauses – 'she gets upset sometimes and what have you. Gives me something useful to do with myself, mind, cheering her up. Makes me feel like her husband again, rather than this useless old git in a bed and her doing everything.'

'She's magic, isn't she?' says the doctor. 'You've never told me how you two met.'

'At the library in town. She worked there Saturdays on the desk. I used to go in once a fortnight to change my book over and she was so lovely, I made sure it was always a Saturday I went. She's probably why I read books.'

The doctor endeavours to have such conversations, if she can, with every patient approaching the end of their life, in the knowledge that there are hard days ahead for the spouse or the children left behind. She always sends a bereavement card when a patient dies and these exchanges at the bedside often yield something personal and meaningful. It started spontaneously many years ago with patients she knew particularly well, but over time it became clear how much value people place on this small act of kindness. Years later, patients will remember 'that lovely card you sent when Mum passed away', and now the wider practice team has rallied behind it. Every so often, the assistant practice manager will buy twenty cards for the bottom-left-hand drawer of the doctor's desk, or one of the receptionists will say, 'You have remembered, haven't you, to send a card to Mrs So-and-Such?' This last terrible year, there have been weeks when the drawer of bereavement cards has run empty. Yet the value of this lies deeper even than the crisis of the moment. The doctor's come to realize that this simple gesture on behalf of the practice does everyone good: the patients, their families, but also the practice staff and the wider community. It consolidates trust in the institution of the surgery and forges fellowship over the generations. It is a quiet statement that 'Here in the valley, this is what we do, this is how we are.'

The doctor now mentions the stout wedge of a paperback novel on the dying man's bedside table. There's an illustration of an eagle on the cover, its talons flexed above a storm-tossed ocean. She's not read that one, she says, but she's read another by the same author, which she liked.

'His first one, was it?' he says. She nods. 'Yes, I read that too. Years ago. Upset the wife the other day though, when I started this one. She says to me, "You can't read that. You might not finish it." And then she realized what she'd said and got very sad, poor thing. But I said, "Don't worry, love. It's not that good."'

THE FOREST THAT towers above the river seems to the untrained eye a natural wilderness, but the appearance is deceptive. These woodlands have been managed by humans over many centuries. Indeed, the valley looks as it does today because people and nature have come together to make it so, and its future depends upon that ongoing relationship.

It's easy to look back on the days when Dr John cared for his patients here and be similarly deceived. For the now apparently heroic medical care provided by him and old-school general practitioners all over the country was there (as one eminent GP recently wrote in a letter to the medical press) not by design, but by default, by nature if you will. Doctors like Berger's Sassall, often working single-handed, were responsible for their patients 24 hours a day, and, barring holidays, every day of the year. That was the way it was, like it or not. In his case, it was a fortuitous collision of temperament and circumstance that gave the valley their fortunate man. It was not the application of a designated framework such as those that appear in contemporary medical discourse: 'relationship-based care', 'the therapeutical relationship', 'person-centred care' or 'relational continuity'. Today, if you deem these things to be desirable, you cannot simply wait for a hero and hope. You have to design a system to include them.

Yet for Dr John and his contemporaries, the continuity, and the trusting relationships that flowed from it, were as organic as the dog roses and celandine that grew in the woods below his house. To an extent, this remains true of the doctor today. The character of this community and the landscape that shapes it affords her more opportunities than many to build and sustain trust, to find purpose and inspiration in her patients' stories over time and across generations. And all of it in this valley that she loves. This is the raw material with which she has worked to become the kind of doctor she is. Nature and design have come together, perhaps. If you ask what makes her a fortunate woman, this is the answer she gives.

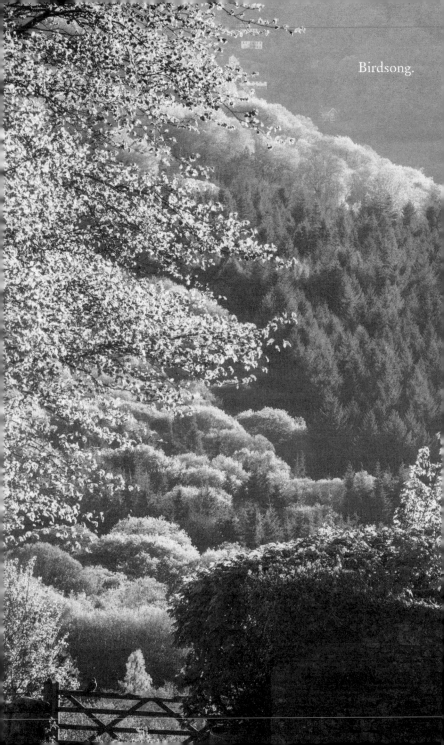

Birdsong.

After the longest of winters comes spring. The budding woods weave a tapestry of trilling, cooing, warbling, twittering, chirruping, whistling back and forth, calling near and far. It is a music so spatial in its acoustics that if she too could take to the wing, she could surely fly around inside the sound, like a sparrow in a great cathedral. The valley beneath is returning to life.

Outside her white stone cottage, the woods full of light, the doctor leans her bike against the garden wall and looks out. Many of her patients are now vaccinated, and around half of her daily appointments are again face to face. She has two new partners, both women, and this year she will start to train new GPs at the practice. Who knows what lies ahead, but she is beginning to feel hopeful again. She crouches down next to her bike to peer into a hole in the wall where a stone came loose a few weeks ago. Inside, there is now a nest. New life, she thinks.

Epilogue

IT IS A CURIOUS experience to narrate a life that is still in train, to tell the story of someone whose story is far from over. Towards the end of *A Fortunate Man*, John Berger wrestles with exactly this as he poses a series of unanswerable questions as to the fundamental value of Dr Sassall's work. 'We in our society,' he writes, 'do not know how to acknowledge, to measure the contribution of an ordinary working doctor. By measure I do not mean *calculate* according to a fixed scale, but, rather, *take the measure of*.'

More than half a century since those words were written of another ordinary doctor working in this bowl of woods and water and meadows and sky, the question remains as enigmatic as ever. For myself, I am unvexed by the impossibility of finding a definitive answer. The doctor's work described in this book, like that of Sassall before her, concerns something as fluid and ever-changing as the river that flows between their two houses. It is about the practice and process of care, the nature of trust and the ebb and flow of the relationships that sustain it. But the reason to narrate her life, I have learned, is that the innate humanity of this work, so taken for granted in Dr John's day, is not as timeless as it once seemed. If we do not measure its value, both *calculate* and *take the measure of*, then we risk losing it altogether. That is why there is something in the stories here to fight for.

So perhaps it was the landscape that brought us together,

the doctor and me, this valley, the woods, the river, our home. Perhaps it was the book that had slipped behind my family bookcase all those years ago, the Penguin paperback of *A Fortunate Man*, priced at 45 new pence or 9 shillings. Perhaps it was my mother, my beloved mother, who had bought the book in the first place and then mislaid it. She died a few months into my work with the doctor, but one of our last conversations at the care home in those final, clouded days concerned the works of John Berger, which she admired greatly and recollected with uncanny clarity for one who was so ill. I told her about my hopes for this book and she told me that Berger would be a hard act to follow. She was right.

Or perhaps it was ultimately the fortunate man himself, that troubled, brilliant doctor who gave more than half his life to this valley, and who then, from beyond the grave, introduced me to his successor, the fortunate woman.

And that seems a fitting place to end.

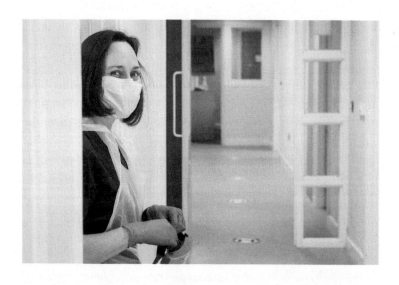

Acknowledgements & Sources

Heartfelt thanks to my editor, George Morley, and my agent, Patrick Walsh, for believing in this book from the very beginning; also to the photographer, Richard Baker, and the book's designers, inside and out, Lindsay Nash and Lucy Scholes, for helping me to tell the story with pictures as well as words. The wider team at Picador, Salma Begum, Kate Berens, Laura Carr, Marissa Constantinou, Bryony Croft, Camilla Elworthy, Philip Gwyn Jones, Simon Rhodes and Giacomo Russo, have been superb throughout, as have John Ash, Margaret Halton and Rebecca Sandell at Pew Literary. I am also immensely grateful to the Royal Literary Fund and The Society of Authors for their generosity and support.

From conversations about medicine, art or life (and sometimes all three) to feedback on early drafts or assistance with the ethics, sensitivities and practicalities of the writing process, I am indebted to the following people, who have shaped this book in manifold ways: Elizabeth Allen-Williams, Jonathan Axe, Sarah Aspinall, Sarah Bagnall, Helen & Ashton Beale, Mandy & Steve Bennett, Jill Berryman, Sandra Bidmead, Rosie Bishop, Andy Brown, Joan Brown, Kathryn Brown, Ruth Brown, Dr Tony Calland, Maria Church, Jonathan Cope, Bill Creswick, Karen Dack, Roger Deeks, Sandra Down, Lee Elmer, Carol & Simon Eskell, Gary Field, Louise & Andrew Frankel, Harry

Josephine Giles, Christine Green, Jason Griffiths, Kathryn Hagg, Dr Lois Harris, Robin Harris, Rosalind Mary Hawken, Beth Hawkins, Dr Martyn Hewett, Caroline & Charles Hopkinson, Kate Humble, Dr Jim Huntley, Elizabeth & Kevin Karney, Frank Kemp, Dr Vivienne Kent, Adrian Levy, Colin Lewis, Simone McCartney, John Meechan, Maxine Morland, Karen Newman, Fiona O'Sullivan, Dr Helen Penny, Lyndsay Price, Cathy Scott-Clark, Val Smith, Tim Stephens, Lucy Tang, John Topp, Amanda Vaughan, Nicolas Webb, Tessa Williams, Ursula Williams, Gemma Wood, George Woodward.

While the documentary process has provided the spine of my research, numerous books and medical papers have also proved indispensable. The lodestar, of course, is John Berger & Jean Mohr's *A Fortunate Man* (Penguin, 1967), reissued in 2015 by Canongate, with an insightful new introduction by Gavin Francis. Other Berger works to which I've frequently turned include *Another Way of Telling* (Bloomsbury, 2016), *The Shape of a Pocket* (Bloomsbury, 2001), *Photocopies* (Bloomsbury, 1996) and *Understanding a Photograph*, edited and introduced by Geoff Dyer (Penguin Classics, 2013). I am also indebted to the woodland ecologist George Peterken for his extraordinary body of scholarship on the landscape and to the community histories collected by William J. Creswick and Julian Wimpenny.

The lion's share of my sources concern medicine, including Michael Balint's classic, *The Doctor, his Patient & the Illness* (Churchill Livingstone, 1957), *The Doctor's Communication Handbook* by Peter Tate (Radcliffe Medical Press, 1994), Iona Heath's monograph 'The Mystery of General Practice' (The Nuffield Provincial Hospital Trust, 1995), Roger Neighbour's *The Inner Consultation* (Petroc Press, 1996), *The New Consultation* by David Pendleton et al. (OUP, 2003), and *Using CBT in General Practice* by Lee David (Scion, 2006), which prompted the doctor's revelation on p. 128. Days and weeks were spent sifting through hundreds of papers and articles chiefly from the *British Medical Journal*, *The Lancet* and the *British Journal of General Practice*, many of which influenced the ideas here and several of which are referred to within the text. These include: Cerel, J. et al., 'How many people are exposed to suicide? Not six', *Suicide and Life-Threatening Behavior* 2018 (on p. 115); Eby, D., 'Empathy in general practice: its meaning for patients and doctors', *BJGP* 2018; Friedemann Smith, C. et al., 'Understanding the role of GPs' gut feelings in diagnosing cancer in primary care: a systematic review and meta-analysis of existing evidence', *BJGP* 2020 (on p. 110); Greenhalgh, T. et al., 'Evidence based medicine: a movement in crisis?', *BMJ* 2014; Haslam, D., 'Risky business: the challenge of being a GP', NICE blog (15 December 2014); Hodes, S. et al., 'If general practice fails, The NHS fails', BMJ Blog (14 May 2021) (on p. 216); Jones, R., 'General practice in the years ahead: relationships will matter more than ever', *BJGP* 2021; Marshall, M., 'The power of trusting relationships in general practice', *BMJ* 2021; Marshall, M. et al., 'The power of relationships: what is relationship-based care and why is it important?', Royal College of General Practitioners Report 2021 (on p. 80); McWhinney, I. R., 'The Importance of Being Different', The William Pickles Lecture 1996; Pereira Gray, D. et al., 'The worried well', *BJGP* 2020 (on p. 126); Pereira Gray, D. et al., 'Covid 19: a fork in the road for general practice', *BMJ* 2020 (on pp. 191–2); Pereira Gray, D. et al., 'Continuity of care with doctors – a matter of life and death? A systematic review of continuity of care and mortality', *BMJ* 2018 (on p. 143); Sandvik, H. et al., 'Continuity in general practice as predictor of mortality, acute hospitalisation, and use of out-of-hours care: a registry-based observational study in Norway', *BJGP* 2022 (on p. 143); Sidaway-Lee, K. et al., 'A method for measuring